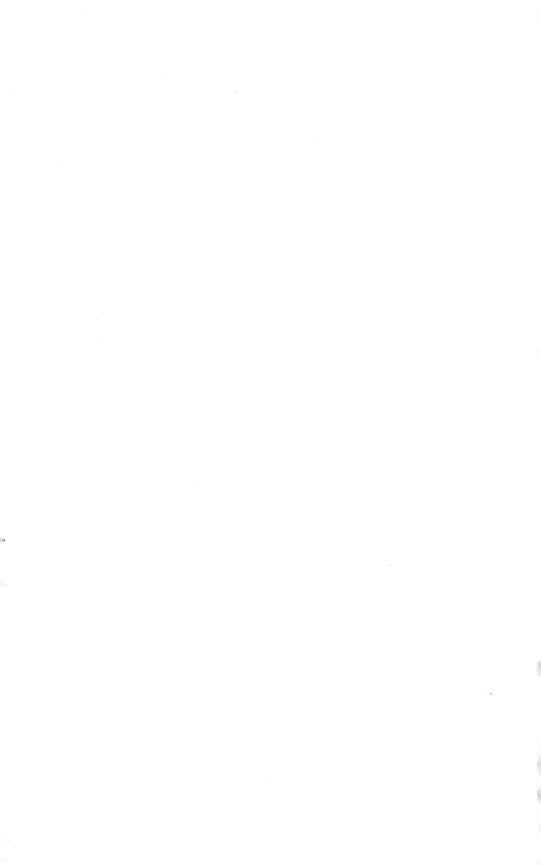

Sommario

GLUTEN-FREE DIET

Fast and Fuss-Free Recipes for Busy People on a Gluten-Free Diet

Miky Morales

All rights reserved.

Disclaimer

The information contained i is meant to serve as a comprehensive collection of strategies that the author of this eBook has done research about. Summaries, strategies, tips and tricks are only recommendation by the author, and reading this eBook will not guarantee that one's results will exactly mirror the author's results. The author of the eBook has made all reasonable effort to provide current and accurate information for the readers of the eBook. The author and it's associates will not be held liable for any unintentional error or omissions that may be found. The material in the eBook may include information by third parties. Third party materials comprise of opinions expressed by their owners. As such, the author of the eBook does not assume responsibility or liability for any third party material or opinions. Whether because of the progression of the internet, or the unforeseen changes in company policy and editorial submission guidelines, what is stated as fact at the time of this writing may become outdated or inapplicable later.

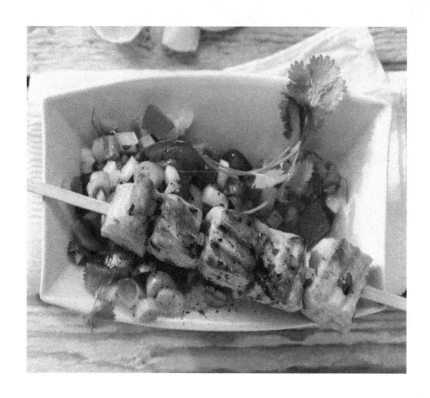

INTRODUCTION
GLUTEN FREE DIET

Gluten is a type of adhesive protein found in most types of grain. The gluten content in wheat is particularly high. Wheat has been cultivated for centuries in such a way that firstly the yield and secondly the gluten content is particularly high.

Because gluten is the magic ingredient in the food industry. It is used as a stabilizer, thickener, gelling agent, flavor carrier, flavoring agent and coloring agent. In particular, gluten ensures that bread and rolls are easy to cut and do not fall apart.

Therefore, gluten is used in almost every industrially manufactured food product. And not only that: Gluten can even be found in medicines, toothpaste and cosmetic products. As a result, it is not so easy at first to completely avoid gluten.

Gluten-free diet as a solution

A strictly gluten-free diet is currently the only therapy that guarantees optimal health for people with celiac disease. The solution for celiac disease is to permanently avoid all foods that are made from gluten-containing grains or contain gluten. Even the smallest traces of gluten can cause histological damage, so special care is required. People with celiac disease must therefore pay particular attention to the selection of their food.

GLUTEN INTOLERANCE OR NON-CELIAC GLUTEN SENSITIVITY

Less hazardous to health, but nonetheless uncomfortable for those affected, is non-celiac gluten sensitivity, i.e., gluten intolerance, which does not express itself as an autoimmune disease, but primarily as an allergy. It causes symptoms similar to those of celiac disease, but has less drastic effects on the health of those affected. There are fewer clear figures for this because non-celiac gluten sensitivity is difficult to prove.

Ultimately, however, the following applies: For people with celiac disease, there is no alternative to a gluten-free diet and for people with gluten intolerance, it is the way to better well-being

The following is a list of those foods that contain or may contain gluten:

Foods containing gluten:

- Grains such as wheat, rye, barley, oats, spelled, green spelled, einkorn, emmer, kamut and products made from them
- Flour, semolina, pearl barley, starch, cereal flakes, muesli
- Pasta, noodles, bread, rolls, baguette, flatbread
- Gnocchi, dumplings, dumplings
- Breadcrumbs and breaded products such as B. breaded meat, breaded fish, breaded cheese
- Meat loaf, meatballs and other minced meat products
- Seitan and products that contain seitan
- Pizza
- Lots of ready meals

- Cakes, pies, puff pastry pieces, yeast pastries
- Cookies, granola bars
- Ice cream cones
- Pretzel sticks, snacks
- Beer and malt beer

The next list should include those products that MAY contain gluten. Here it would make sense - at least if you really want to or have to live completely gluten-free - if you would contact the manufacturer before buying or consuming it.

Hidden gluten:

- Ready-made sauces (including seasoned sauces such as soy and fish sauce), ready-made dressings, ready-made soups
- Medicines, toothpaste, and cosmetic products such as lip balm sticks
- Flavors, colors, stabilizers, thickeners, gelling agents, flavor enhancers
- Edible play dough
- French fries
- Croquettes, potato pancakes
- Dairy products with fruit preparations
- Some reduced fat products
- Cream cheese preparations with herbs
- Sausage and sausages
- Scrambled eggs in restaurants or hotels
- Pudding, ice cream, nut nougat cream
- Chips, flips and other nibbles
- chocolate

- Ketchup, mustard and seasoned sauces such as soy sauce, fish sauce and others
- Spice mixes
- Fashion drinks, lemonades
- Flavored tea or coffee

Add additives to cocoa powder

We have also put together more information on hidden gluten sources for you here: Nine hidden gluten sources.

However, so that you are not so shocked and don't think that you can't eat anything anymore, the following is the positive list with all those products / foods that are gluten-free:

Gluten-free foods:

- Rice, wild rice, corn, millet, buckwheat, amaranth, quinoa and products made from all of these grains and pseudo-grains (e.g., flour, flakes, pops)
- nuts
- Oil seeds (linseed, sesame, pumpkin seeds, sunflower seeds, etc.)
- legumes
- fruit and vegetables
- Salads (be careful with ready-made dressings)
- Potatoes and potato starch
- Chestnuts and products made from them (e.g., chestnut flour, chestnut flakes)
- Plantain flour, soy flour, teff flour, chickpea flour, coconut flour, hemp flour, lupine flour, almond flour
- milk and milk products

- Vegetable oils other than wheat germ oil
- Meat, fish, seafood
- Eggs
- Tofu and soy milk
- Coconut and coconut products (coconut flour, coconut oil, coconut blossom sugar, coconut butter, coconut flakes, etc.)
- Honey and many alternative sweeteners such as maple syrup, agave syrup, apple syrup, rice syrup, yavon as syrup or yacon as powder etc. (barley malt better not)
- pure spices and herbs (be careful with mixtures)
- pure fruit juices, water, tea (not flavored)
- pure cocoa powder
- Wine and champagne

Gluten-free binders: potato starch, rice flour, corn starch, kudzu, arrowroot starch, locust bean gum, gua gum

BENEFITS OF THE GLUTEN-FREE DIET

If you now eat gluten-free, you automatically have the advantage that in future you will not only protect your body from gluten, but also from all the chemical additives that are contained in most ready-made meals.

The easiest way to switch to a gluten-free diet is to start by cooking and baking everything freshly at home. In this way you always know exactly what is really in your food and quickly get a feel for what you can order outside of your home, i.e., in restaurants or hotels, and what better not.

There are now entire shelves in supermarkets, drug stores and health food stores with gluten-free ready-made products such as pizza, bread, rolls and much more. But for the beginning it is advisable to bake and cook yourself in order to get to know the alternative possibilities of gluten-free cuisine.

In addition, the gluten-free finished products off the shelf are gluten-free, but that is often the only criterion. The typical chemical food additives are still included. It may also contain additional substances that are supposed to mimic the properties of the missing gluten.

GLUTEN-FREE RECIPES

RICOTTA PANCAKES WITH APRICOTS

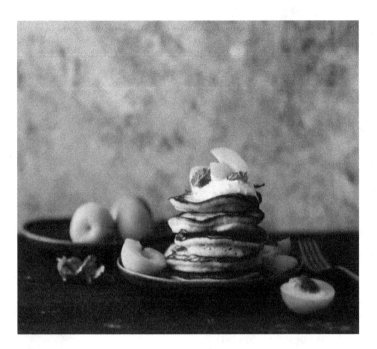

Preparation:

15 minutes

Calories:

499 kcal

Nutritional values

1 serving contains

(proportion of the daily requirement in percent)

- Calories499 kcal   (24%)
- protein 19 g   (19%)
- fat   23 g   (20%)
- carbohydrates 52 g   (35%)
- added sugar   5.3 g   (21%)
- Fiber   2.8 g   (9%)

ingredients for 1 portion

- 80 g ricotta
- 1 egg
- 3 tbsp lemon juice
- 1 tsp honey
- 40 g buckwheat flour
- ½ tsp baking powder
- 1 tsp coconut oil
- 2 apricots
- 3 tbsp yogurt (3.5% fat)
- 1 stem mint

preparation

Kitchen appliances

1 bowl, 1 whisk, 1 pan, 1 spatula, 1 knife, 1 work board

Preparation steps

1. Mix the ricotta with the egg, lemon juice and honey until smooth. Add buckwheat flour and baking powder and mix into a thick batter. Heat coconut oil in a pan and add a large tablespoon of batter to each pan, bake on medium heat for 1 minute, turn and continue baking from the other side. Do this for about 5 pancakes.
2. In the meantime, wash the apricots, halve and cut into wedges. Stir the yogurt until creamy. Wash the mint, shake dry and pick off the leaves. Stack the pancakes on a plate, place the yogurt and apricot wedges on top and serve garnished with mint.

Vanilla yogurt with apricots

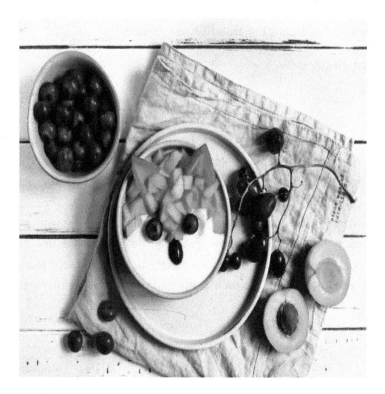

Preparation:

15 minutes

Calories:

145 kcal

Nutritional values

1 serving contains

(proportion of the daily requirement in percent)

- Calories 592 kcal   (28%)
- protein 21 g   (21%)
- fat   23 g   (20%)
- carbohydrates 74 g   (49%)
- added sugar   0 g   (0%)
- Fiber   16.7 g   (56%)

ingredients for 2 portions

- 250 g yogurt (3.5% fat)
- 1 tsp linseed oil
- 1 pinch vanilla powder
- 2 apricots
- 4th banana slices
- 4th blueberries
- 2 red grapes

preparation

Kitchen appliances

1 knife, 1 work board

Preparation steps

1. Mix yoghurt with vanilla powder and linseed oil and divide into two bowls.
2. Wash fruit and pat dry. Halve the apricots and stone them. Cut ears from one apricot half, cut the rest into small cubes.
3. Place a fox face with the apricot cubes on the yoghurt, leaving free space for your chin and cheeks. Assemble eyes from the banana slices and blueberries. Place the grapes as a nose on the yogurt and finally place the ea

HONEY SKYR WITH NUTS

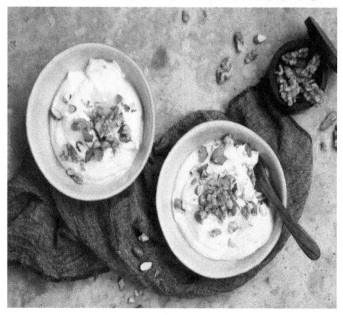

Preparation:

5 min

Calories:

373 kcal

Nutritional values

1 serving contains

(proportion of the daily requirement in percent)

- Calories 373 kcal   (18%)
- protein 30 g   (31%)
- fat   21 g   (18%)
- carbohydrates 15 g   (10%)
- added sugar   7.5 g   (30%)
- Fiber   2 g   (7%)

ingredients for 2 portions

- 400 g skyr
- 1 tbsp honey (alternatively maple syrup)
- 1 pinch vanilla powder
- 1 handful walnut kernels (25 g)
- 1 handful almond kernels (25 g; unpeeled)
- 2 tsp linseed oil

preparation

Kitchen appliances

2 small bowls, 1 knife, 1 work board

Preparation steps

1. Mix the skyr with honey and vanilla. Roughly chop the walnuts and almonds.
2. Divide the skyr into two bowls, pour the nuts over them and drizzle 1 teaspoon of linseed oil over each. Serve and enjoy Skyr.

Vegetable and lentil stew with peas

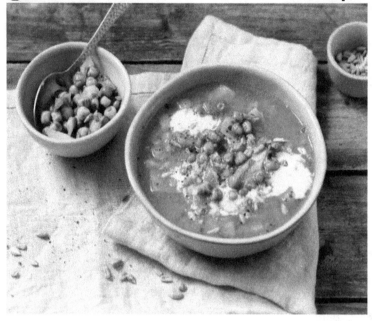

Preparation:

25 min

Calories:

592 kcal

Nutritional values

1 serving contains

(proportion of the daily requirement in percent)

- Calories592 kcal   (28%)
- protein 21 g   (21%)
- fat   23 g   (20%)
- carbohydrates 74 g   (49%)
- added sugar   0 g   (0%)
- Fiber   16.7 g   (56%)

ingredients for 2 portions

- 5 g ginger tuber
- 1 shallot
- 1 sweet potato
- 100 g celery root
- 2 tbsp olive oil
- 80 g red lenses
- 1 tsp harissa paste
- 1 tbsp tomato paste
- ½ tsp curry powder
- 600 ml vegetable broth
- salt
- pepper
- 4 tbsp coconut milk
- 2 pieces spring onions
- 150 g frozen pea
- 2 tsp sunflower seeds

preparation

Kitchen appliances

1 work board, 1 small knife, 1 pot

Preparation steps

1. Peel and chop the ginger and shallot. Clean and peel the sweet potato and celery and cut into small cubes.
2. Heat 1 tablespoon of oil in a saucepan, sauté the ginger, shallot, sweet potato and celery over a medium heat for 5 minutes. Add lentils, harissa, tomato paste and curry powder and sauté for 4 minutes.
3. Pour the vegetable stock, season with salt and pepper and let the soup simmer for about 15 minutes. Then stir in 2 tablespoons of coconut milk.
4. At the same time, clean, wash and chop the spring onions. Heat the remaining oil in a pan, fry the onion, peas and sunflower seeds for 5 minutes. Fill the soup into two bowls, drizzle with the remaining coconut milk and top with the peas.

Grilled salmon skewers with fennel and tomato salsa

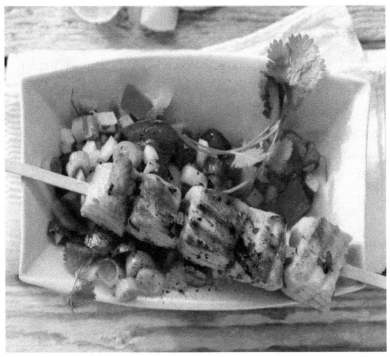

Preparation:

40 min

ready in 1 h

Calories:

225 kcal

Nutritional values

1 serving contains

(proportion of the daily requirement in percent)

- Calories 225 kcal   (11%)
- protein 19 g   (19%)
- fat   14 g   (12%)
- carbohydrates 4 g   (3%)
- added sugar   1 g   (4%)
- Fiber   2.5 g   (8th %)

ingredients for 4 portions

- 200 g fully ripe tomatoes
- 2 spring onions
- 150 g fennel bulb (1 fennel bulb)
- 1 red chilli pepper
- 3 stems coriander
- 1 lime
- 3 tbsp olive oil
- salt
- sugar
- 400 g salmon fillet without skin
- 1 dried chili pepper
- Pepper

preparation

Kitchen appliances

1 bowl, 1 small bowl, 1 work board, 1 large knife, 1 small knife, 1 tablespoon, 1 wooden spoon, 1 grill pan, 4 wooden skewers

Preparation steps

1. Wash, quarter and core the tomatoes, removing the stalks.
2. Divide the pulp into 1 cm cubes.
3. Wash and clean the spring onions and cut into rings 1/2 cm thick.
4. Wash the fennel, cut in half, remove the stalk and finely dice the tuber.
5. Halve the fresh chilli lengthways, remove the core, wash and finely chop.
6. Wash the coriander, shake dry and chop the leaves.
7. Squeeze the lime.
8. Mix the finely chopped ingredients with 1 tablespoon each of lime juice and oil. Season with salt and a pinch of sugar. Before serving, chill and let steep for at least 30 minutes.
9. Cut the salmon fillet into 12 equal cubes.
10. Crumble the dried chilli pepper, mix with the pepper and the remaining oil and pour over the salmon. Let it steep for 15 minutes (marinate).
11. Lightly salt the salmon cubes and place on 4 wooden skewers. Heat a grill pan and grill the skewers all around for 4-5 minutes. Place the salmon skewers and salsa on a plate and serve with lime wedges if desired.

Kheer Indian rice pudding

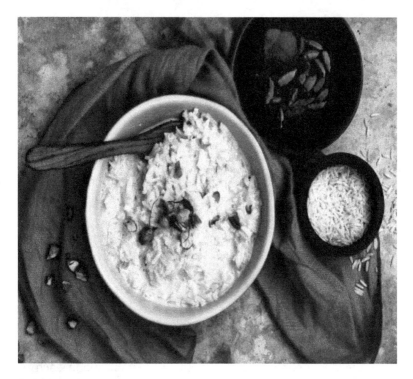

Preparation:

10 min

ready in 50 min

Calories:

323 kcal

Nutritional values

1 serving contains

(proportion of the daily requirement in percent)

- Calories323 kcal   (15%)

- protein 11 g   (11%)
- fat   12 g   (10%)
- carbohydrates 43 g   (29%)
- added sugar   5 g   (20%)
- Fiber   1.7 g   (6%)

ingredients for 4 portions

- 125 g basmati rice
- 750 ml milk (3.5% fat)
- 1 pinch saffron
- 4 tsp raw cane sugar
- 4th green cardamom pods
- 1 clove
- ½ tsp cinnamon powder (ceylon)
- 1 handful almonds (with skin)
- 2 tsp rose water (as required)
- 1 tbsp pistachio nuts

preparation

Kitchen appliances

1 small pot, 1 knife, 1 measuring cup

Preparation steps

1. Put rice in a bowl and soak in cold water for 30 minutes. Strain and wash with cold water.
2. Put the milk, sugar and saffron in a saucepan. Press on the cardamom pods and add to the milk with the clove and cinnamon and bring to the boil.
3. As soon as the milk starts to boil, stir in rice and simmer covered for about 20 minutes over low heat. Stir occasionally to prevent the rice from sticking and burning.
4. Meanwhile, finely chop the almonds and add to the rice. If necessary, stir in the rose water into the kheer, season to taste and divide into bowls. Top with coarsely chopped pistachios and enjoy cold or warm.

Quinoa salad

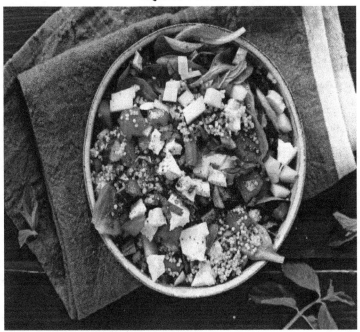

Preparation:

1 h

Calories:

409 kcal

Nutritional values

1 serving contains

(proportion of the daily requirement in percent)

- Calories 409 kcal (19%)
- protein 15 g (15%)
- fat 16 g (14%)
- carbohydrates 50 g (33%)
- added sugar 0 g (0%)

- Fiber   8.9 g   (30%)

ingredients for 4 portions

- 200 g quinoa
- 1 mango
- 1 cucumber
- 3 tomatoes
- 1 red pepper
- 150 g lamb's lettuce
- 1 red onion
- 2 stems mint
- 150 g feta (45% fat in dry matter)
- 1 tbsp olive oil
- 1 tbsp apple cider vinegar
- salt
- pepper

preparation

Kitchen appliances

1 saucepan, 1 sieve, 1 knife, 1 work board, 1 bowl

Preparation steps

1. Rinse the quinoa with cold water, bring to the boil in a saucepan with twice the amount of water and cook over a low heat for about 10 minutes. In the meantime, peel the mango, cut from the stone and dice the pulp. Clean, wash and cut the cucumber, tomatoes and peppers. Wash the lamb's lettuce and spin dry. Peel and chop the onion. Wash the mint, shake dry, pluck the leaves and cut into strips. Dice the feta.

2. Drain the quinoa, drain and place in a bowl. Add the mango, cucumber, tomatoes, bell pepper, lamb's lettuce, onion, mint and feta and mix. Season the salad with olive oil, apple cider vinegar, salt and pepper.

Burrito bowl

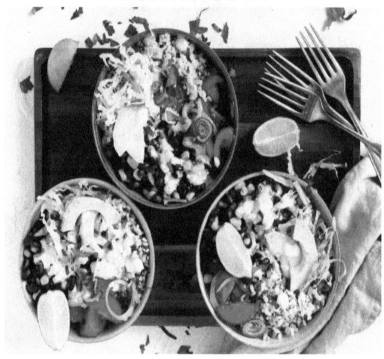

Preparation:

45 min

Calories:

388 kcal

Nutritional values

1 serving contains

(proportion of the daily requirement in percent)

- Calories 388 kcal   (18%)
- protein 9 g   (9%)
- fat   17 g   (15%)
- carbohydrates 48 g   (32%)
- added sugar   0 g   (0%)
- Fiber   6 g   (20%)

ingredients for 4 portions

- 200 g whole grain rice
- salt
- 1 federal government parsley (20 g)
- 2 organic limes
- 100 g black beans (can; drained weight)
- 100 g corn (can; drained weight)
- 1 green chilli pepper
- 2 tbsp olive oil
- pepper
- 200 g cherry tomato
- 1 small red onion
- 1 lettuce heart
- 1 avocado
- ½ clove of garlic
- 200 g greek yogurt

preparation

Kitchen appliances

1 saucepan, 1 lemon squeezer, 1 sieve, 1 hand blender

Preparation steps

1. Put rice in a saucepan with twice the amount of salted water, bring to a boil and cook covered over medium heat for 25 minutes.

2. In the meantime, wash the parsley and shake dry. Set aside 1 small handful, chop the remaining parsley. Squeeze the juice of 1 lime. Fluff the rice and let it evaporate. Fold in the chopped parsley and 1 tbsp lime juice.

3. Drain the beans and corn in a colander, wash and drain. Clean and wash the chilli pepper, remove the seeds and finely chop. Mix the beans, corn and chilli with 1 tablespoon of olive oil and season with salt and pepper.

4. Clean, wash and quarter the cherry tomatoes. Peel and halve the onion and cut into rings. Mix tomatoes and onion rings with 1 tablespoon of oil and 1 teaspoon of lime juice, season with salt and pepper.

5. Clean, wash and cut the lettuce into fine strips. Halve the avocado, remove the core and remove the pulp with a spoon. Cut diagonally into strips. Peel the garlic and purée finely with the yogurt, remaining parsley, a little lime juice, salt and pepper. Wash the remaining lime with hot water, rub dry and cut into 4 wedges.

6. Divide the parsley rice, bean and corn mix, tomatoes and lettuce into 4 bowls and serve with avocado strips and yoghurt dressing. Serve garnished with remaining parsley leaves and lime wedges.

Cucumber, radish and tomato salad

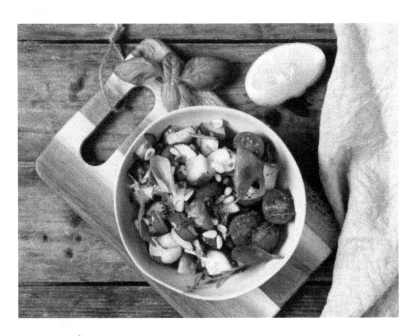

Preparation:

10 min

Calories:

199 kcal

Nutritional values

1 serving contains

(proportion of the daily requirement in percent)

- Calories 199 kcal   (9%)
- protein 5 g   (5%)
- fat   16 g   (14%)

- carbohydrates   8 g   (5%)

ingredients for 4 portions

- 1 ½ cucumbers
- 1 federal government radish
- 1 federal government rocket (80 g)
- 250 g cherry tomatoes
- 4 tbsp olive oil
- 3 tbsp lemon juice
- 1 tsp mustard
- 1 tsp honey
- salt
- pepper
- 40 g pine nuts
- ½ fret basil

preparation

Kitchen appliances

1 work board, 1 large knife, 1 salad bowl

Preparation steps

1. Clean and wash the cucumber and radishes. Cut the cucumber into cubes and the radishes into thin slices. Wash the rocket and shake dry. Wash tomatoes and cut in half.
2. For the dressing, whisk the oil with lemon juice, mustard and honey, season with salt and pepper. Mix the cucumbers, radishes, tomatoes and rocket and mix with the dressing.
3. Roast pine nuts in a pan without fat for 3 minutes over medium heat. Wash the basil, shake dry and pick off the leaves. Serve the salad sprinkled with pine nuts and basil.

Spring risotto with green asparagus and radishes

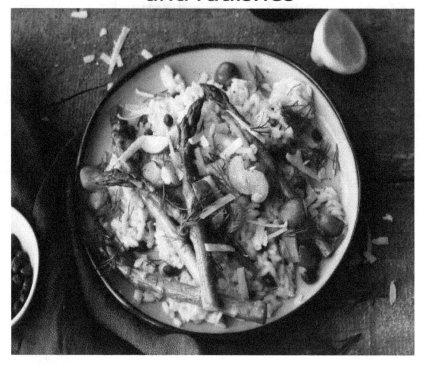

Preparation:

30 min

Calories:

575 kcal

Nutritional values

1 serving contains

(proportion of the daily requirement in percent)

- Calories575 kcal   (27%)
- protein 21 g   (21%)
- fat   20 g   (17%)
- carbohydrates 76 g   (51%)
- added sugar   0 g   (0%)

ingredients for 2 portions

- ½ red onion
- 2 tbsp olive oil
- 180 g risotto rice
- 2 tsp capers
- 650 ml vegetable broth
- 60 g parmesan
- pepper
- 1 splash
- lemon juice
- 400 g green asparagus
- ½ fret radish
- salt
- ½ fret dill

preparation

Kitchen appliances

1 saucepan, 1 knife, 1 work board, 1 pan, 1 grater

Preparation steps

1. Peel half an onion and cut into strips. Heat 1 tablespoon of olive oil in a saucepan, sauté onion and risotto rice for 1 minute over medium heat. Add capers and deglaze with a little vegetable stock. Gradually add the vegetable stock for about 20 minutes, stirring occasionally, until the rice has completely absorbed the liquid.

2. Grate the parmesan and stir half into the risotto. Season with pepper and lemon juice and set aside with the lid closed.

3. In the meantime, clean and wash the asparagus and radishes. Cut off the woody ends of the asparagus and quarter the radishes. Heat the rest of the oil in a pan and fry the vegetables over a medium heat for 3 minutes while turning and season with salt. Wash the dill, shake dry and roughly chop.

4. Arrange the risotto on plates, pour the vegetables on top and serve sprinkled with the rest of the parmesan and dill.

Brussels sprouts and cashew soup

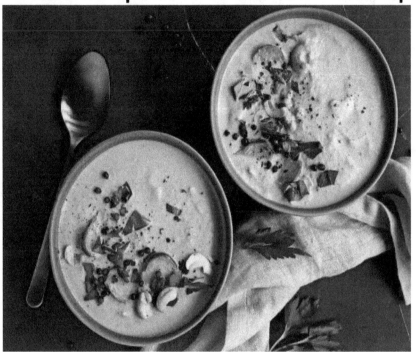

Preparation:

20 min

ready in 4 h 40 min

Calories:

451 kcal

Nutritional values

1 serving contains

(proportion of the daily requirement in percent)

- Calories 451 kcal   (21%)
- protein 19 g   (19%)
- fat   27 g   (23%)
- carbohydrates 32 g   (21%)
- added sugar   0 g   (0%)
- Fiber   10.7 g   (36%)

ingredients for 2 portions

- 110 g cashew nuts
- 300 g brussels sprouts
- 500 ml vegetable broth
- 5 dates (without stone)
- 1 organic lemon
- 1 handful herbs (5 g; e.g., parsley)
- 1 pinch himalayan salt
- pepper
- pink pepper berries

preparation

Kitchen appliances

1 hand blender, 1 saucepan, 1 knife, 1 lemon squeezer

Preparation steps

1. Soak 100 g cashew nuts in 200 ml water for at least 4 hours. Then process into a cream with a mixer.
2. In the meantime, clean and wash the Brussels sprouts, put them in a saucepan with the vegetable stock and cook over a medium heat for 15–20 minutes. Then drain the Brussels sprouts and set aside a few florets. Gradually add the remaining cabbage with the cashew cream and 200 ml water and the dates until the desired consistency is achieved and puree to a creamy soup.
3. Squeeze the lemon. Wash herbs, shake dry and chop. Season the soup with lemon juice, salt and pepper and add the Brussels sprouts set aside. Arrange the soup in bowls and sprinkle with the remaining cashew nuts, pink pepper berries and herbs.

Vegetarian pizza soup

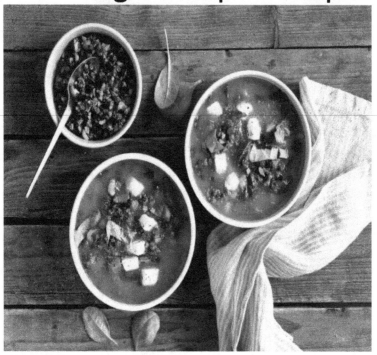

Preparation:

45 min

Calories:

467 kcal

Nutritional values

1 serving contains

(proportion of the daily requirement in percent)

- Calories467 kcal   (22%)
- protein 21 g   (21%)
- fat   37 g   (32%)
- carbohydrates 14 g   (9%)
- added sugar   0 g   (0%)
- Fiber   8.9 g   (30%)

ingredients for 4 portions

- 300 g brown mushrooms
- 1 red onion
- 2 garlic cloves
- 1 yellow pepper
- 1 red pepper
- 100 g baby spinach
- 250 g mozzarella (45% fat in dry matter)
- 4 tbsp hazelnut kernels
- 4 tbsp olive oil
- 500 g strained tomatoes (glass)
- 500 ml vegetable broth
- salt
- pepper
- 2 tsp dried oregano
- 1 tsp dried basil
- 1 tsp paprika powder
- 2 tsp soy sauce

preparation

Kitchen appliances

1 knife, 1 small coated pan, 1 saucepan

Preparation steps

1. Clean the mushrooms, cut them into very small cubes and spread them out on a baking sheet. Let dry for about 30 minutes.
2. In the meantime, peel the onion and garlic, cut the onion into strips and chop the garlic. Clean, wash, halve the peppers, remove the seeds and cut into cubes. Clean and wash the spinach, shake dry and roughly chop, put about a handful aside for the garnish. Drain the mozzarella and cut into small cubes.
3. Roughly chop the hazelnuts and roast them in a pan over medium heat for about 3–5 minutes, remove from the pan and set aside.
4. Heat 2 tablespoons of olive oil in a saucepan, sauté the onions and garlic over a medium heat. Pour tomatoes and broth and simmer for about 10 minutes. Season the pizza soup with salt, pepper, oregano and basil. Then add the paprika, spinach and three quarters of the mozzarella and stir in.
5. Heat the rest of the olive oil in the pan and fry the mushroom cubes in it for about 5 minutes and season with paprika powder, soy sauce and pepper. Then mix with hazelnuts and add to the pizza soup. Sprinkle with the remaining spinach and mozzarella and serve.

Lentil noodles with pesto and Brussels sprouts

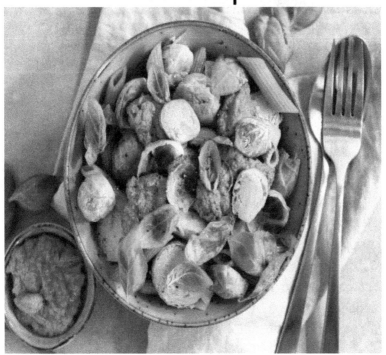

Preparation:

30 min

Calories:

531 kcal

Nutritional values

1 serving contains

(proportion of the daily requirement in percent)

- Calories 531 kcal   (25%)
- protein 28 g   (29%)
- fat   29 g   (25%)
- carbohydrates 39 g   (26%)
- added sugar   0 g   (0%)
- Fiber   12.1 g (40%)

ingredients for 4 portions

- 500 g brussels sprouts
- salt
- 250 g lentil noodles
- 1 clove of garlic
- 80 g dried tomato in oil (drained)
- 50 g parmesan in one piece (30% fat in dry matter)
- 30 g pine nuts (2 tbsp)
- 8 tbsp olive oil
- ½ organic lemon (zest and juice)
- pepper
- 5 g basil leaves (1 handful)

preparation

Kitchen appliances

1 grater, 1 hand blender

Preparation steps

1. Clean, wash and halve the Brussels sprouts. Cook the florets in salted boiling water for 5 minutes. Then drain, rinse and drain.
2. At the same time cook the pasta in boiling salted water for 8 minutes according to the instructions on the packet; then drain and drain.
3. Meanwhile, cut the dried tomatoes into small pieces. Grate the parmesan. Roast the pine nuts in a hot pan without fat over medium heat for 3 minutes.
4. Finely puree the tomatoes, parmesan, pine nuts, oil and 3–4 tablespoons of water with a hand blender and season with salt, pepper, lemon zest and juice. Wash the basil and shake dry. Mix pasta with Brussels sprouts and serve with pesto and basil.

Stuffed sweet potato with eggplant and feta

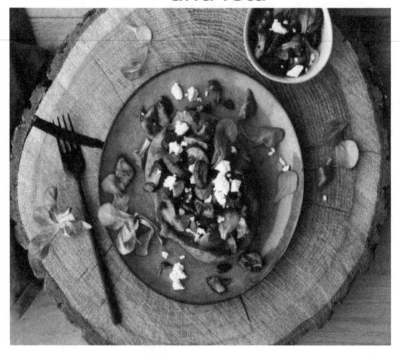

Preparation:

20 min

ready in 1 h 10 min

Calories:

644 kcal

Nutritional values

1 serving contains

(proportion of the daily requirement in percent)

- Calories644 kcal   (31%)
- protein 18 g   (18%)
- fat   34 g   (29%)
- carbohydrates 66 g   (44%)
- added sugar   0 g   (0%)
- Fiber   11.7 g (39%)

ingredients for 2 portions

- 500 g sweet potatoes (2 small sweet potatoes)
- 1 aubergine
- 3 tbsp olive oil
- 4th sun-dried tomatoes
- 20 g pumpkin seeds
- ½ tsp hot pink paprika powder
- 1 pinch chilli flakes
- ½ tsp ground cumin
- 1 pinch ground cardamom
- salt
- pepper
- 1 handful
- lamb's lettuce
- 100 g feta

preparation

Kitchen appliances

1 baking dish, 1 knife, 1 work board, 1 pan, 1 bowl

Preparation steps

1. Wash the sweet potatoes, pat dry, cut lengthways and insert several times with a fork. Place in a baking dish and bake in a preheated oven at 200 ° C (fan oven: 180 ° C; gas: level 3) for about 60 minutes.
2. In the meantime, wash the eggplant and cut it into cubes. Heat 1 tbsp olive oil in a pan and fry the eggplant cubes over medium heat for 5 minutes. Cut the dried tomatoes into strips and roughly chop the pumpkin seeds. Mix the spices with the remaining oil, mix with the aubergine cubes, season with salt and pepper.
3. Wash the lamb's lettuce and spin dry. Crumble the feta. Let the baked sweet potatoes cool down a little, open a little, mash the pulp with a fork, season with salt and pepper. Fill with eggplant mixture, feta and lamb's lettuce and serve.

Bowl with potatoes, cucumber, avocado and feta

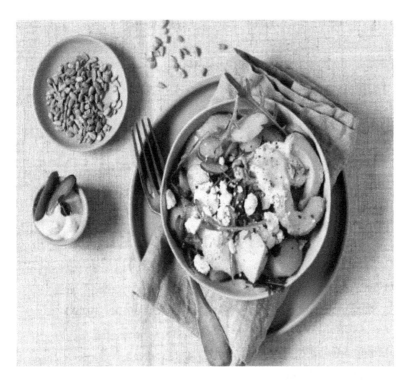

Preparation:

25 min

Calories:

483 kcal

Nutritional values

1 serving contains

(proportion of the daily requirement in percent)

Calories483 kcal   (23%)

protein 14 g   (14%)

fat   27 g   (23%)

carbohydrates 43 g   (29%)

added sugar   0 g   (0%)

Fiber   9.3 g   (31%)

ingredients for 2 portions

- 400 g waxy potatoes
- salt
- ½ cucumber
- ½ fret radish
- 1 handful
- arugula
- 1 avocado
- 4 pieces pickled cucumber (with 1 tbsp cucumber stock)
- 4 tbsp yogurt (3.5% fat)
- 1 tbsp linseed oil
- 1 branch marjoram
- pepper
- 50 g feta
- 2 tsp sunflower seeds

preparation

Kitchen appliances

1 saucepan, 1 work board, 1 small knife, 1 salad bowl, 1 bowl

Preparation steps

1. Peel and wash the potatoes and cook for 15 minutes in salted boiling water. Then drain, rinse in cold water and let drain.
2. Meanwhile, clean and wash the cucumber and radishes and cut into thin slices. Wash the rocket and shake dry. Halve 2 pickles lengthways and cut into slices; dice the rest. Halve the avocado, remove the stone, lift the pulp out of the skin and cut into strips.
3. For the dip, wash the marjoram, shake dry and chop the leaves. Then mix the yogurt, oil, marjoram, diced cucumber and cucumber stock, season with salt and pepper.
4. Crumble the feta. Cut the potatoes into slices and mix with the cucumber, radish and rocket. Pour ingredients into bowls, add avocado, sprinkle with feta and sunflower seeds and drizzle with the dip.

Sweet potatoes with asparagus, eggplant and halloumi

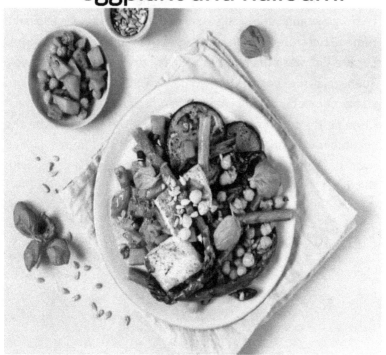

Preparation:

45 min

Calories:

789 kcal

Nutritional values

1 serving contains

(proportion of the daily requirement in percent)

- Calories 789 kcal   (38%)
- protein 32 g   (33%)

- fat 50 g (43%)
- carbohydrates 53 g (35%)
- added sugar 1 g (4%)
- Fiber 10 g (33%)

ingredients for 4 portions

- 1 aubergine
- 9 tbsp olive oil
- chilli flakes
- salt
- pepper
- 2 sweet potatoes
- 1 red chilli pepper
- 2 tbsp sunflower seeds
- 1 federal government green asparagus
- 4 tbsp lemon juice
- 200 g chickpeas (can; drop weight)
- ½ fret basil
- ½ fret lemon balm
- 1 tsp mustard
- ½ tsp turmeric powder
- 1 tsp honey
- 300 g halloumi

preparation

Kitchen appliances

1 work board, 1 large knife, 1 coated pan

Preparation steps

1. Clean, wash and slice the eggplant. Heat 2 tablespoons of oil in a pan and fry the aubergine slices on both sides for 5–7 minutes on

a medium heat and season with chilli flakes, salt and pepper. Remove from pan and set aside.

2. Meanwhile, peel the sweet potato and cut into cubes. Halve the chilli lengthways, remove the core, wash and cut into slices. Heat 1 more tablespoon of oil in the pan and fry the sweet potato cubes for 10 minutes. Add 1 tbsp sunflower seeds and chilli slices and season with salt and pepper. Also set aside.

3. At the same time wash the asparagus, cut off the woody ends, if necessary, peel the lower third of the stalks. Heat 1 tablespoon of oil in a pan, fry the asparagus in it for 5 minutes over medium heat. Deglaze with 1 tbsp lemon juice, add 2 tbsp water and cook covered for another 3 minutes.

4. At the same time rinse the chickpeas and drain them. Wash the basil and lemon balm, shake dry and chop. Mix the chickpeas with half of the herbs and 1 tablespoon of oil and season with salt and pepper.

5. For the dressing, whisk the remaining oil with the rest of the lemon juice, mustard, turmeric and honey, season with salt and pepper and mix in the remaining herbs.

6. Cut the halloumi into slices and fry in a hot pan on both sides for 5 minutes over medium heat until golden.

7. To serve, arrange sweet potatoes and aubergine slices on plates, pour chickpeas, asparagus and halloumi over them and drizzle with the dressing. Sprinkle with the leftover sunflower seeds.

Lentil salad with spinach, rhubarb and asparagus

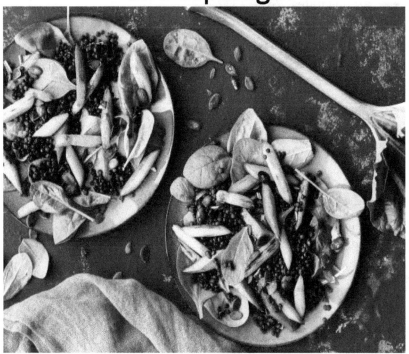

Preparation:

25 min

ready in 35 min

Calories:

324 kcal

Nutritional values

1 serving contains

(proportion of the daily requirement in percent)

- Calories324 kcal   (15%)
- protein 19 g   (19%)
- fat   16 g   (14%)
- carbohydrates   26 g   (17%)
- added sugar   2.6 g   (10%)
- Fiber   13.2 g (44%)

ingredients for 2 portions

- 100 g beluga lentils
- 2 tbsp olive oil
- salt
- 250 g white asparagus
- 100 g rhubarb
- 1 tsp honey
- 50 g baby spinach (2 handfuls)

preparation

Kitchen appliances

1 pan, 1 saucepan, 1 sieve, 1 knife, 1 work board, 1 peeler, 1 salad spinner

Preparation steps

1. Bring the beluga lentils to the boil with three times the amount of water. Cook over medium heat for about 25 minutes. Drain, rinse and drain. Mix with 1 tbsp olive oil and a pinch of salt. In the meantime, wash, clean, peel the asparagus and cut diagonally into pieces. Wash and clean the rhubarb and cut into pieces.
2. Heat 1 tablespoon of olive oil in a pan and fry the asparagus for about 8 minutes over medium heat, swirling occasionally. Then add rhubarb and honey and fry and salt for another 5 minutes. Wash the spinach and spin dry. Roughly chop the pumpkin seeds.
3. Arrange the spinach with lentils, asparagus and rhubarb on two plates and serve sprinkled with pumpkin seeds.

Healthy green shot

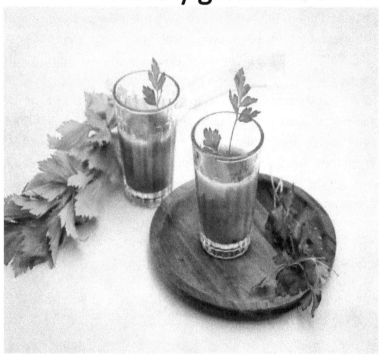

Preparation:

15 minutes

Calories:

33 kcal

Nutritional values

1 serving contains

(proportion of the daily requirement in percent)

- Calories33 kcal (2%)
- protein 0 g (0%)
- fat   0 g (0%)
- carbohydrates 7 g   (5%)
- added sugar   0 g   (0%)
- Fiber   2 g   (7%)

ingredients for 25 portions

- 2 pears
- 3 green apples (e.g. granny smith)
- 3 poles celery
- 60 g organic ginger
- 1 federal government parsley (20 g)
- 3 kiwi fruit
- 2 limes
- 1 tsp turmeric

preparation

Kitchen appliances

1 work board, 1 small knife, 1 lemon squeezer, 1 juicer

Preparation steps

1. Wash pears, apples, celery, ginger and parsley and cut into pieces. Halve the kiwi fruit and remove the pulp with a spoon. Halve the limes and squeeze out the juice.
2. Put pears, apples, kiwis, celery, ginger and parsley in the juicer and squeeze out the juice.

3. Mix freshly squeezed juice with lime juice and season with turmeric. Serve mixture immediately as shots or freeze in portions.

Pea soup with feta and dill

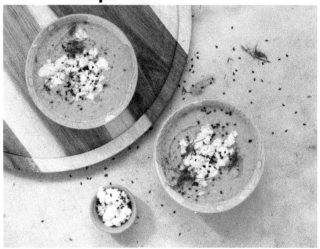

Preparation:

15 minutes

Calories:

533 kcal

Nutritional values

1 serving contains

(proportion of the daily requirement in percent)

- Calories 533 kcal   (25%)
- protein 21 g   (21%)
- fat   40 g   (34%)
- carbohydrates   23 g   (15%)
- added sugar   0 g   (0%)
- Fiber   8.8 g   (29%)

ingredients for 2 portions

- 1 shallot
- 1 clove of garlic
- 2 tbsp olive oil
- 300 g peas (frozen)
- 200 ml vegetable broth
- 4 stems dill
- 100 g feta
- 100 g whipped cream
- salt
- pepper
- chilli flakes
- 1 tsp black sesame

preparation

Kitchen appliances

1 pot, 1 hand blender

Preparation steps

1. Peel the shallot and garlic. Heat 1 tablespoon of oil in a saucepan, sauté shallots and garlic for 3 minutes over medium heat. Then add the peas and cook for another 3 minutes.
2. Then pour in the vegetable stock and simmer for about 5 minutes. In the meantime, wash the dill, shake it dry and finely pluck it. Crumble the feta.
3. Then pour the cream and use a hand blender to finely puree the soup with half of the dill. Season the pea soup with salt, pepper and chili flakes. Fill into two bowls, sprinkle with the rest of the dill, feta and sesame seeds and drizzle with the rest of the oil.

Chia yogurt with clementine puree

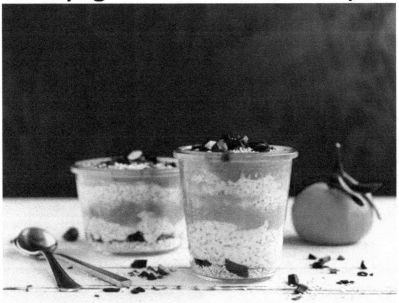

Preparation:

10 min

ready in 15 min

Calories:

446 kcal

Nutritional values

1 serving contains

(proportion of the daily requirement in percent)

- Calories446 kcal   (21%)
- protein 14 g   (14%)
- fat   23 g   (20%)
- carbohydrates 44 g   (29%)
- added sugar   3.3 g   (13%)
- Fiber   9.3 g   (31%)

ingredients for 2 portions

- 300 g lactose-free yogurt (1.5% fat)
- 30 g chia seeds
- 1 tsp whole cane sugar
- 2 clementines
- 1 banana
- 1 pinch
- cinnamon
- 30 g dark chocolate
- 30 g hazelnuts
- 5 g amaranth pops (2 tbsp)

preparation

Kitchen appliances

1 bowl, 1 stand mixer, 1 knife, 1 work board

Preparation steps

1. Mix the yogurt with the chia seeds and whole cane sugar and set aside.

2. Peel the clementines and divide into fillets. Peel the banana and place in the blender with the clementines. Season with cinnamon and puree everything finely.
3. Finely chop the dark chocolate and hazelnuts.
4. Layer the yoghurt-chia mix and fruit puree alternately in two glasses, ending with a layer of puree. Serve sprinkled with chocolate, hazelnuts and puffed amaranth

Grilled chicken

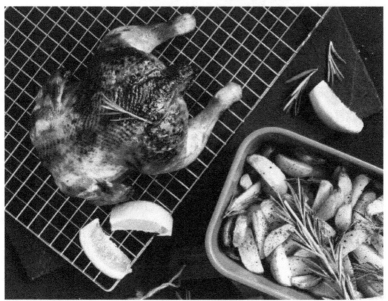

Preparation:

1 h 15 min

Calories:

619 kcal

Nutritional values

1 serving contains

(proportion of the daily requirement in percent)

- Calories619 kcal   (29%)
- protein 56 g   (57%)
- fat   24 g   (21%)
- carbohydrates 42 g   (28%)
- added sugar   2.8 g   (11%)
- Fiber   3.5 g   (12%)

ingredients for 4 portions

- 1 ½ kg roast chicken (1 roast chicken)
- salt
- pepper
- 1 tbsp honey
- 4 tbsp soy sauce
- 1 tsp curry
- 8th shallots
- 2 garlic bulbs
- 600 g small potatoes
- 1 federal government rosemary

preparation

Kitchen appliances

1 grill skewer, 1 aluminum grill tray

Preparation steps

1. Wash the chicken, pat dry and season with salt and pepper on the inside. Put on a skewer. Mix the honey, soy sauce and curry together and brush the chicken with it.
2. Peel the shallots and cut the garlic in half crosswise.
3. Wash the potatoes and cut into wedges. Place in a grill tray with rosemary sprigs, salt and pepper. Grill the chicken and place the

vegetables underneath. Grill for about 1 hour. Stir the vegetables several times.

Salmon cutlet on kohlrabi salad with fennel and watercress

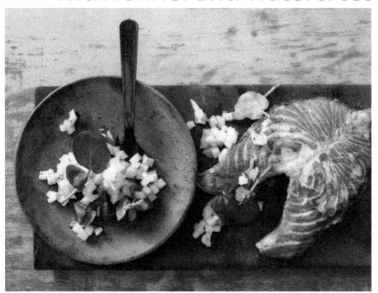

Preparation:

25 min

Calories:

243 kcal

Nutritional values

1 serving contains

(proportion of the daily requirement in percent)

- Calories 243 kcal   (12%)
- protein 27 g   (28%)
- fat   10 g   (9%)
- carbohydrates 9 g   (6%)
- added sugar   3 g   (12%)
- Fiber   5.5 g   (18%)

ingredients for 2 portions

- 1 small shallot
- 200 g small kohlrabi (1 small kohlrabi)
- 200 g small fennel bulb (1 small fennel bulb)
- 50 g watercress
- 200 g thin salmon cutlet (2 thin salmon cutlets)
- pepper
- 4 tsp olive oil
- salt
- 3 tbsp apple cider vinegar
- ½ tsp mustard
- 1 tsp liquid honey

preparation

Kitchen appliances

1 work board, 1 whisk, 1 coated pan, 1 small bowl, 1 bowl, 1 tablespoon, 1 teaspoon, 1 small knife, 1 fine sieve, 1 kitchen paper, 1 spatula, 1 salad servers

Preparation steps

1. Peel and finely dice shallot. Put in a fine sieve and scald with boiling water.
2. Peel and clean the kohlrabi, wash and clean the fennel. Cut both into small cubes.
3. Wash watercress and shake dry, cut into bite-sized pieces as desired.
4. Rinse the salmon cutlets, pat dry, season with pepper.
5. Heat 2 teaspoons of oil in a coated pan. Fry the salmon cutlets on each side for 3-4 minutes and lightly salt.
6. Mix the vinegar, mustard, honey and remaining oil in a small bowl. Mix the kohlrabi, fennel, shallot and watercress with the sauce. Serve with the salmon cutlets.

Cucumber and radish salad with feta

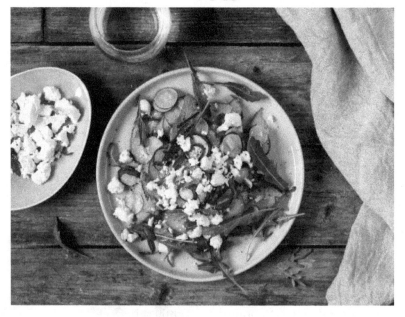

Preparation:

15 minutes

Calories:

273 kcal

Nutritional values

1 serving contains

(proportion of the daily requirement in percent)

- Calories 273 kcal   (13%)
- protein 10 g   (10%)
- fat   23 g   (20%)
- carbohydrates 7 g   (5%)
- added sugar   1 g   (4%)
- Fiber   2.8 g   (9%)

ingredients for 4 portions

- 1 ½ cucumbers
- 1 federal government radish
- 1 federal government rocket (80 g)
- 4th gherkins
- 200 g feta
- 4 tbsp olive oil
- 3 tbsp lemon juice
- 1 tsp mustard
- 1 tsp honey
- salt
- pepper

preparation

Kitchen appliances

1 work board, 1 large knife, 1 salad bowl

Preparation steps

1. Clean and wash the cucumber and radishes and cut into thin slices. Wash the rocket and shake dry. Halve the pickles lengthways and cut into slices. Crumble the feta.
2. For the dressing, whisk the oil with lemon juice, mustard and honey, season with salt and pepper. Mix the cucumber, radish and pickled cucumber slices and mix with the dressing. Place on the plate and sprinkle with the feta and rocket.

Vegan tomato spread

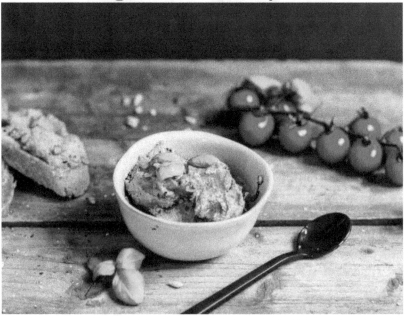

Preparation:

15 minutes

Calories:

139 kcal

Nutritional values

1 serving contains

(proportion of the daily requirement in percent)

- Calories 139 kcal   (7%)
- protein 5 g   (5%)
- fat   10 g   (9%)
- carbohydrates 8 g   (5%)
- added sugar   0 g   (0%)
- Fiber   1.9 g   (6%)

ingredients for 6 portions

- 100 g dried tomato in oil
- 100 g sunflower seeds
- 3 tbsp olive oil
- 1 handful basil
- 1 pinch raw cane sugar
- salt
- pepper

preparation

Kitchen appliances

1 hand blender, 1 sieve, 1 tall vessel

Preparation steps

1. Drain the tomatoes slightly in a colander and cut roughly. Put the tomatoes in a tall container and puree them together with the sunflower seeds, olive oil and 4 tablespoons of water.

2. Wash the basil, shake dry and finely chop the leaves. Add the basil to the tomato spread and stir in.
3. Season the tomato spread with raw cane sugar, salt and pepper. The tomato spread can be kept airtight in the refrigerator for 4-5 days.

Cream of carrot soup with nut croutons

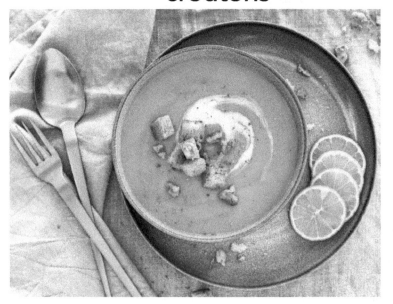

Preparation:

20 min

ready in 35 min

Calories:

367 kcal

Nutritional values

1 serving contains

(proportion of the daily requirement in percent)

- Calories367 kcal   (17%)
- protein 7 g   (7%)
- fat   15 g   (13%)
- carbohydrates 51 g   (34%)
- added sugar   0 g   (0%)
- Fiber   10 g   (33%)

ingredients for 4 portions

- 500 g carrots
- 400 g sweet potatoes
- 1 tart apple
- 1 onion
- 2 garlic cloves
- 30 g ginger
- 3 tbsp olive oil
- 400 ml coconut milk (can)
- 3 tsp curry powder
- 1 pinch cinnamon
- salt
- pepper
- 2 wholemeal bread slices
- 3 tbsp walnut kernels
- 2 tbsp lime juice

preparation

Kitchen appliances

1 knife, 1 saucepan, 1 hand blender

Preparation steps

1. Wash and chop the carrots. Wash, peel and cut the sweet potato and apple. Peel and dice the onion, garlic and ginger.
2. Heat 1 tablespoon of oil in a saucepan. Add onion, garlic and ginger and simmer over medium heat for 2-3 minutes. Add carrots, sweet potatoes and apple and sauté for 2 minutes.
3. Stir coconut milk and set aside 4 tablespoons for the garnish. Pour the carrot mix up with the remaining coconut milk and 500 ml of water. Season carrot soup with curry, cinnamon, salt and pepper, bring to the boil and simmer covered for 15 minutes over a low heat.
4. In the meantime, dice the bread and roughly chop the walnuts. Heat the remaining oil in a pan. Add bread cubes and walnuts and fry for 3–4 minutes until crispy.
5. Puree the carrot soup finely. Season to taste with salt, pepper and lime juice. Garnish the carrot soup with the coconut milk that was set aside and sprinkle with nut croutons.

Apple compote

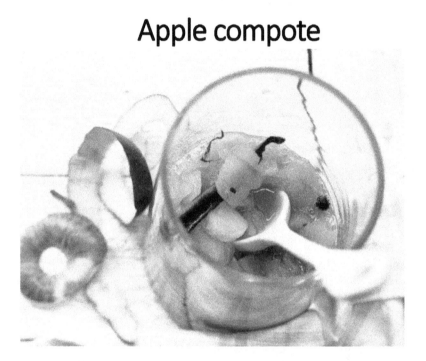

Preparation:

25 min

ready in 2 h 25 min

Calories:

200 kcal

Nutritional values

1 serving contains

(proportion of the daily requirement in percent)

- Calories 200 kcal (10%)
- protein 1 g (1 %)
- fat 0 g (0%)
- carbohydrates 48 g (32%)
- added sugar 11.3 g (45%)
- Fiber 4 g (13%)

ingredients for 4 portions

- 800 g tart apples (4 tart apples)
- 50 g coconut blossom sugar
- 1 pole cinnamon
- 3 allspice grains
- 200 ml

preparation

Kitchen appliances

1 saucepan, 1 measuring cup, 1 work board, 1 large knife, 1 wooden spoon, 1 peeler, 1 core cutter

Preparation steps

1. Peel the apples and core them with a core cutter or halve the apples and cut out the core with a knife.
2. Quarter the apples and cut into slices or roughly cubes.
3. Melt coconut blossom sugar in a saucepan over medium heat until light brown (caramelize).
4. Add cinnamon and allspice. Pour in the apple juice, bring to the boil while stirring until the caramel has dissolved. Add the apples

and cook covered for about 12 minutes over a low heat, stirring occasionally. Then pour the apple compote into a bowl and let it cool down.

5.

Mushroom salad with garlic, zucchini and feta

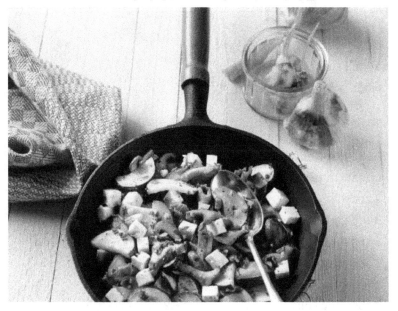

Preparation:

30 min

ready in 40 min

Calories:

258 kcal

Nutritional values

1 serving contains

(proportion of the daily requirement in percent)

- Calories258 kcal   (12%)
- protein 17 g   (17%)
- fat   18 g   (16%)
- carbohydrates 7 g   (5%)
- added sugar   0 g   (0%)
- Fiber   5.1 g   (17%)

ingredients for 6 portions

- 600 g mixed fresh mushrooms chanterelles, champignons, porcini mushrooms
- 2 zucchini
- 3 red garlic cloves
- 1 shallot
- 3 spring onions
- 1 federal government chives
- 2 tbsp olive oil
- 2 tbsp white balsamic vinegar
- Salt pepper from the mill
- 200 g diced feta

preparation

Kitchen appliances

1 knife, 1 work board, 1 pan

Preparation steps

1. Clean the mushrooms and cut into slices or pieces. Wash the zucchini, clean, cut in half and also cut into slices. Peel and finely dice the garlic and onion. Wash the spring onions and chives, shake dry and cut into rings or rolls.
2. Heat the oil in a pan and sauté the mushrooms for 3–4 minutes while swirling. Add the zucchini, onion, garlic and spring onions and fry briefly. Remove from heat and let cool down briefly. Mix the vinegar with the chives, season with salt and pepper and mix into the salad together with the diced feta. Serve lukewarm.

Steamed fish fillet on bed of vegetables

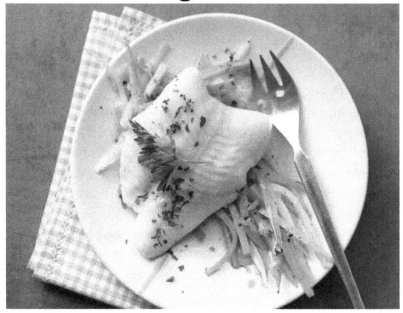

Preparation:

25 min

Calories:

100 kcal

Nutritional values

1 serving contains

(proportion of the daily requirement in percent)

- Calories100 kcal (5%)
- protein 13 g (13%)
- fat 2 g (2%)
- carbohydrates 5 g (3%)
- added sugar 0 g (0%)
- Fiber 6 g (20%)

ingredients for 1 portion

- 1 shallot
- ½ tuber fennel
- 60 g small carrots (1 small carrot)
- 3 tbsp classic vegetable broth
- salt
- pepper
- 70 g pangasius fillet (preferably organic pangasius)
- 2 stems flat leaf parsley
- ½ small lime

preparation

Kitchen appliances

1 work board, 1 small knife, 1 peeler, 1 tablespoon, 1 coated pan with lid, 1 wooden spoon, 1 large knife, 1 lemon squeezer, 1 pallet or spatula

Preparation steps

1. Peel and finely dice shallot.
2. Clean and wash the fennel and carrot, peel the carrot thinly. Cut both vegetables into narrow sticks.
3. Heat the stock in a coated pan. Add shallot, fennel and carrot and cook for about 3 minutes. Season to taste with salt and pepper.
4. Rinse the fish fillet, pat dry, lightly salt and place on the vegetables. Cover and cook over a low heat for 8-10 minutes.
5. In the meantime, wash the parsley, shake dry, pluck the leaves and finely chop with a large knife.
6. Squeeze half a lime and drizzle the juice over the fish to taste. Pepper to taste, sprinkle with parsley and serve.

Grilled fennel

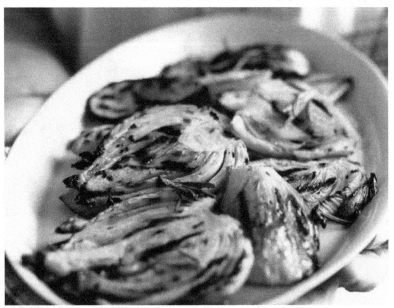

Preparation:

15 minutes

Calories:

92 kcal

Nutritional values

1 serving contains

(proportion of the daily requirement in percent)

- Calories92 kcal (4%)

- protein 4 g   (4%)
- fat   6 g   (5%)
- carbohydrates 8 g   (5%)
- added sugar   0 g   (0%)
- Fiber   5 g   (17%)

ingredients for 4 portions

- 4th fennel bulbs
- 2 tbsp olive oil
- 1 branch rosemary
- salt
- pepper from the grinder

preparation

Kitchen appliances

1 knife, 1 work board, 1 grill

Preparation steps

1. Clean and wash the fechel and cut it lengthways into slices. Place on a table or charcoal grill and grill for 2-3 minutes on each side.
2. Tear apart the rosemary and place between the hot slices of fennel. Drizzle the fennel with olive oil and season with salt and pepper. Serve immediately.

Mexico bowl with rice, corn, beans and guacamole

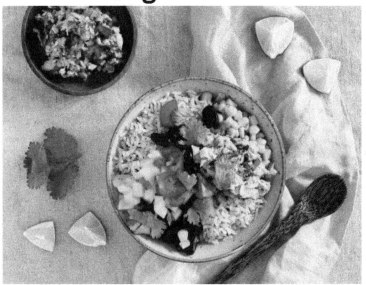

Preparation:

25 min

Calories:

482 kcal

Nutritional values

1 serving contains

(proportion of the daily requirement in percent)

- Calories482 kcal   (23%)
- protein 14 g   (14%)
- fat   16 g   (14%)
- carbohydrates 69 g   (46%)
- added sugar   0 g   (0%)
- Fiber   14.6 g   (49%)

ingredients for 4 portions

- 250 g rice-fit brown rice
- iodized salt with fluoride
- 2 avocados
- 2 organic limes
- ½ red onion
- 1 chilli pepper
- ½ fret coriander (10 g)
- pepper
- 250 g cherry tomatoes
- 1 yellow pepper
- 200 g corn (can; drained weight)
- 200 g kidney beans (can; drained weight)

preparation

Kitchen appliances

1 saucepan, 1 knife, 1 sieve

Preparation steps

1. For the rice, bring 500 ml water with almost ½ teaspoon salt to the boil. Add the rice-fit natural rice and stir once. Simmer over low heat in a closed pot for 8-10 minutes until the rice has absorbed the water. Then loosen the rice briefly in the pot and stir it a few more on the switched off stove and then let it cool for 10 minutes.

2. In the meantime, for the guacamole, halve the avocados, remove the stone, lift the pulp out of the shell with a spoon, place in a bowl and roughly mash with a fork. Rinse limes with hot and squeeze the juice from one lime. Drizzle the lime juice over the avocado pulp. Peel the onion and dice very finely. Halve the chilli lengthways, remove the core, wash and finely chop. Wash the coriander, shake dry and finely chop the leaves. Mix half of the onion, chilli and ¾ of the coriander greens with the avocado and season with salt and pepper.

3. Wash and quarter the tomatoes. Halve, core, wash and dice the pepper. Rinse the corn and beans in a colander and allow to drain. Then arrange the rice and the prepared ingredients in four bowls. Top with guacamole and sprinkle with the rest of the coriander. Quarter the rest of the lime and serve with the bowl.

Quinoa curd casserole with fruit salad

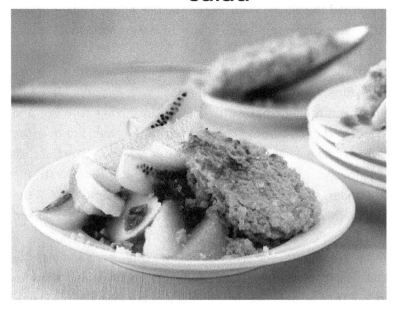

Preparation:

30 min

ready in 1 h 10 min

Calories:

482 kcal

Nutritional values

1 serving contains

(proportion of the daily requirement in percent)

- Calories 482 kcal   (23%)
- protein 27 g   (28%)
- fat   7 g   (6%)
- carbohydrates 73 g   (49%)
- added sugar   10 g   (40%)
- Fiber   7.5 g   (25%)

ingredients for 4 portions

- 150 g quinoa
- 100 ml milk (1.5% fat)
- 400 g oranges (2 oranges; 1 of them organic)
- 2 eggs
- 20 g brown cane sugar (1 tbsp)
- 500 g lowfat quark
- ½ tsp cinnamon
- ½ tsp ground ginger
- liquid sweetener (at will)
- 1 tsp germ oil
- 2 tbsp raisins
- 2 kiwi fruit
- 200 g apples (1 apple)
- 400 g bananas (2 bananas)

preparation

Kitchen appliances

1 sieve, 1 measuring cup, 1 pot with lid, 1 fine grater, 1 tall vessel, 1 hand mixer, 1 tablespoon, 1 teaspoon, 1 wooden spoon, 1 casserole dish (approx. 1.5 l content), 1 brush, 1 work board, 1 small knife, 1 bowl

Preparation steps

1. Put quinoa in a colander, rinse with hot water and drain. Bring to the boil with 200 ml of water and the milk in a saucepan and cook covered over a low heat for 15 minutes. Cover and leave to soak for another 5 minutes on the switched off stove. Then let cool in the open pot.
2. While the quinoa is cooking, wash the organic orange with hot water, rub dry and finely grate about ¼ of the peel.
3. Separate the eggs and place the egg whites in a tall container. Beat with the whisk of the hand mixer until stiff and let the sugar trickle in gradually.
4. Mix the quark and egg yolks with the quinoa. Season with grated orange peel, cinnamon and ginger. Fold in the whipped egg whites and add sweetener to taste.
5. Grease a flat casserole dish (approx. 1.5 l capacity) with the oil and pour in the quinoa quark mixture. Bake in a preheated oven at 200 ° C (convection 180 ° C, gas: level 3) for about 30 minutes.
6. In the meantime, peel both oranges so thick that all white is removed. Cut out the fruit fillets between the separating

membranes and collect the juice in a bowl. Add the orange fillets. Roughly chop the raisins and also add to the bowl.

7. Peel and halve the kiwi fruit and cut into wedges. Wash the apple, rub dry, quarter, core and also cut into fine wedges. Fold both under the orange fillets.

8. Peel the bananas, cut them into slices, add them to the bowl and let everything sit for about 10 minutes. Serve the fruit salad with the quinoa quark bake.

Mixed leaf salads with avocado and shaved pecorino

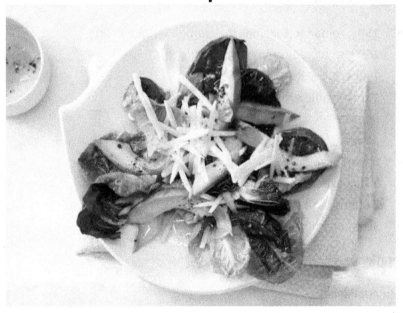

Preparation:

25 min

Calories:

257 kcal

Nutritional values

1 serving contains

(proportion of the daily requirement in percent)

- Calories 257 kcal   (12%)
- protein 3 g   (3%)
- fat   25 g   (22%)
- carbohydrates 3 g   (2%)
- added sugar   1 g   (4%)
- Fiber   2 g   (7%)

ingredients for 4 portions

- 150 g roman lettuce heart (1 roman lettuce heart)
- 150 g small radicchio (1 small radicchio)
- 1 lime
- 1 tbsp maple syrup
- fleur de sel
- pepper
- 6 tbsp olive oil
- 1 ripe avocado
- 2 stems basil
- 30 g pecorino (1 piece)

preparation

Kitchen appliances

1 lemon squeezer, 1 salad spinner, 1 work board, 1 large knife, 1 small knife, 1 tablespoon, 1 coarse grater, 1 small bowl, 1 small whisk, 1 bowl

Preparation steps

1. Clean, wash and spin dry the salads. Slice the leaves as desired and place in a bowl.
2. Halve and squeeze the lime.
3. For the vinaigrette, mix lime juice with maple syrup, a little fleur de sel and pepper. Beat the olive oil with a whisk.
4. Peel and halve the avocado, remove the stone and cut the pulp lengthways into thin slices.
5. Wash the basil, spin dry and pluck the leaves. Cut the leaves into fine strips.
6. Drizzle half of the vinaigrette over the salad. Mix carefully and serve on 4 plates.
7. Pour the remaining salad sauce over the avocado slices and serve the slices with the salad.
8. Pour the basil over it and grate the cheese over it.

Avocado and min ice cream with chocolate

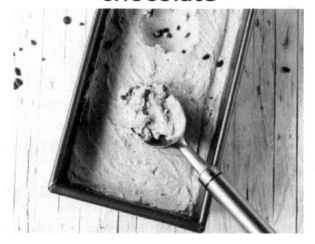

Preparation:

15 minutes

ready in 2 h 15 min

Calories:

368 kcal

Nutritional values

1 serving contains

(proportion of the daily requirement in percent)

- Calories 368 kcal   (18%)
- protein 4 g   (4%)
- fat   31 g   (27%)
- carbohydrates 20 g   (13%)
- added sugar   14 g   (56%)
- Fiber   5.7 g   (19%)

ingredients for 6 portions

- 400 ml coconut milk (can)
- 3 ripe avocados
- 10 g mint (0.5 bunch)
- 2 tbsp lemon juice
- 50 g agave syrup

preparation

Kitchen appliances

1 large bowl, 1 hand mixer, 1 knife, 1 hand blender, 1 box baking pan

Preparation steps

1. Open the coconut milk and spoon out the solid part at the top - do not shake the can beforehand - and place in a large bowl. Beat the firm coconut milk with a hand mixer until frothy and then pour it into a cake or casserole dish.
2. Halve the avocados, remove the pits, remove the pulp and place in a blender. Wash the mint, shake dry and pluck the leaves. Puree the avocado pulp with lemon juice, agave syrup and mint to a creamy and smooth mass.

3. Put the avocado mixture on the frothy coconut cream, sprinkle with chocolate drops and mix the mixture carefully but evenly. The surface of the mass should be relatively smooth.
4. Place cling film on the ice cream mass and press down gently so that there is no air between the film and the ice cream mass. Put the ice in the freezer for at least 2 hours.
5. Let thaw briefly and enjoy.

Sweet potato and radish pan with pomegranate seeds

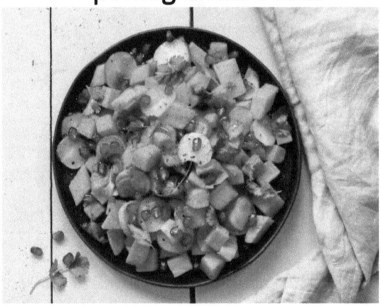

Preparation:

30 min

Calories:

272 kcal

Nutritional values

1 serving contains

(proportion of the daily requirement in percent)

- Calories272 kcal   (13%)
- protein 4 g   (4%)
- fat   4 g   (3%)
- carbohydrates 52 g   (35%)
- added sugar   0 g   (0%)
- Fiber   7.7 g   (26%)

ingredients for 4 portions

- 800 g sweet potatoes (2 pieces)
- 20 g ginger
- 1 federal government radish
- 1 tbsp sesame oil
- ¼ tsp ground cumin
- ¼ tsp ground coriander
- 1 lime
- ½ pomegranate
- 1 federal government coriander green (20 g)
- salt
- pepper

Preparation steps

1. Peel the sweet potatoes and cut into 1–1.5 cm cubes. Peel and chop the ginger. Clean, wash and slice the radishes.
2. Heat the oil in a large non-stick pan. Add ginger and sauté for 1–2 minutes over medium heat. Add the sweet potato cubes and simmer for about 7–8 minutes over medium heat.
3. Add cumin and coriander and simmer for 2 minutes. Then add the radishes and cook for another 2-3 minutes.

4. In the meantime, halve the lime and squeeze out the juice. Halve the pomegranate and remove the stones from the fruit. Wash the coriander, shake dry and remove the leaves.
5. Deglaze sweet potatoes with lime juice and season with salt and pepper. Serve sprinkled with pomegranate seeds and coriander.

Keto vegetable curry with cauliflower rice

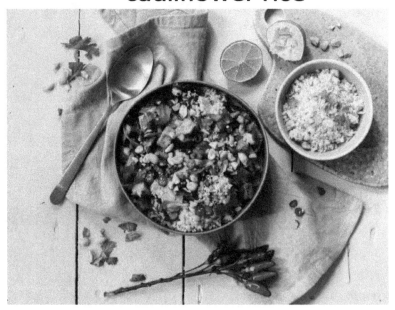

Difficulty:

light

Preparation:

40 min

Calories:

381 kcal

Nutritional values

1 serving contains

(proportion of the daily requirement in percent)

- Calories 381 kcal   (18%)
- protein 14 g   (14%)
- fat   32 g   (28%)
- carbohydrates 9 g   (6%)
- added sugar   0 g   (0%)
- Fiber   5 g   (17%)

ingredients for 4 portions

- 1 shallot
- 1 clove of garlic
- 10 g ginger (1 piece)
- 300 g eggplant (1 eggplant)
- 200 g baby spinach
- 150 g tofu
- 2 tbsp coconut oil
- 1 tsp turmeric powder
- 1 tsp garam masala
- 1 tsp curry powder
- 150 ml vegetable broth
- 300 ml coconut milk
- 2 tbsp lime juice
- salt
- pepper
- 30 g peanut kernel
- 10 g coriander green (0.5 bunch)
- 1 chilli pepper

- 200 g cauliflower
- 1 tbsp peanut oil

preparation

Kitchen appliances

1 knife, 1 work board, 1 salad spinner, 1 pot, 1 food processor, 1 pan

Preparation steps

1. Peel and finely chop shallot, garlic and ginger. Wash and clean the aubergine and cut into cubes. Wash the spinach and spin dry. Drain the tofu and cut into cubes.
2. Heat coconut oil in a saucepan. Sauté shallot, garlic and ginger in it. Add the aubergine cubes and tofu and fry them, then add the turmeric powder, garam masala and curry powder. Add the spinach and let it collapse. Pour the vegetable stock on top and bring to the boil briefly. Pour in coconut milk, then cook over medium heat for about 10 minutes. Season with 1 tbsp lime juice, salt and pepper.
3. In the meantime, roughly chop the peanuts. Wash the coriander, shake dry and also roughly chop. Wash and clean the chilli pepper and cut into fine rings.
4. Wash the cauliflower, cut into florets and chop to the size of a grain of rice in a food processor. Heat the peanut oil in a pan and fry the cauliflower rice over medium heat for about 5 minutes while stirring. Season with the rest of the lime juice, salt and pepper.
5. Divide the cauliflower rice in 4 bowls and top with the keto vegetable curry. Sprinkle everything with peanuts, coriander and chili rings and serve.

Sweet potato toast with hummus and beetroot

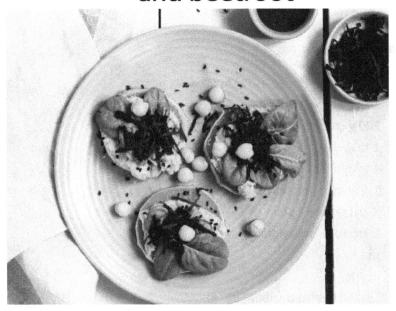

Preparation:

20 min

Calories:

415 kcal

Nutritional values

1 serving contains

(proportion of the daily requirement in percent)

- Calories 415 kcal   (20%)
- protein 13 g   (13%)
- fat   13 g   (11%)
- carbohydrates 61 g   (41%)
- added sugar   0 g   (0%)
- Fiber   11.5 g   (38%)

ingredients for 2 portions

- 300 g sweet potatoes (1 small sweet potato)
- 1 small clove of garlic
- 200 g chickpeas (can; drained weight)
- 1 tbsp olive oil
- 1 tbsp tahini (sesame paste)
- 1 splash lemon juice
- ½ tsp ground cumin
- ½ tsp rose-hot paprika powder
- salt
- pepper
- 1 small beetroot tuber (100 g)
- 40 g baby spinach
- 1 tsp black cumin

preparation

Kitchen appliances

1 hand blender

Preparation steps

1. Peel, wash and cut the sweet potato into 4–6 slices. Bake the slices in a preheated oven at 200 ° C (fan oven 180 ° C; gas: level 3) for about 8–10 minutes.
2. In the meantime, peel the garlic for the hummus. Rinse the chickpeas, drain them and finely puree 150 g chickpeas with garlic, oil, tahini, lemon juice, cumin, paprika powder and 2 tbsp water with a hand blender. Season to taste with salt and pepper.
3. Peel, wash and finely grate the beetroot. Wash the spinach and pat dry.
4. Take the sweet potato slices out of the oven, brush with hummus and top with beetroot and spinach. Serve sprinkled with black cumin.

Stew with various vegetables

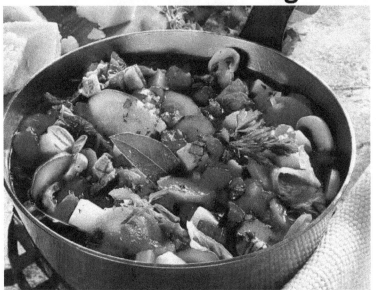

Preparation:

35 min

ready in 50 min

Calories:

126 kcal

Nutritional values

1 serving contains

(proportion of the daily requirement in percent)

- Calories 126 kcal   (6%)
- protein 8 g   (8th %)
- fat   7 g   (6%)
- carbohydrates 7 g   (5%)
- added sugar   0 g   (0%)
- Fiber   5 g   (17%)

ingredients for 4 portions

- 1 onion
- 2 garlic cloves
- 100 g carrots
- 100 g celery root
- 200 g savoy
- 100 g zucchini
- 100 g mushrooms
- 1 federal government basil (20 g)
- ½ fret parsley (10 g)
- 2 branches oregano
- 2 tomatoes
- 1 tbsp olive oil
- 1 l vegetable broth
- 1 bay leaf
- 50 g parmesan
- salt
- pepper

preparation

Kitchen appliances

1 knife, 1 pot, 1 work board

Preparation steps

1. Peel the onion and garlic, chop finely. Peel the carrot and cut into thin slices, clean the celery, peel finely dice, clean the savoy cabbage, wash and cut into wide strips, clean the zucchini, wash and cut into thin slices. Clean the mushrooms, cut into fine leaves. Wash herbs, shake dry and finely chop. Scald tomatoes with hot water, rinse with cold water, peel off the skin, dice finely.
2. Heat the oil in a saucepan, sauté the onion and garlic, deglaze with the broth, add the bay leaf. Add carrots and celery, cook covered for 5 minutes, add savoy cabbage and mushrooms, simmer for another 4 minutes. Add tomatoes and zucchini, simmer for 3 minutes.
3. Grate the parmesan. Before serving, season the stew with vegetables with salt and pepper, sprinkle with herbs and parmesan.

Summer fruit salad

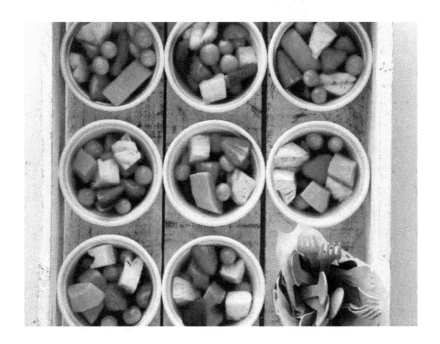

Preparation:

20 min

Calories:

253 kcal

Nutritional values

1 serving contains

(proportion of the daily requirement in percent)

- Calories 253 kcal   (12%)
- protein 4 g   (4%)
- fat   1 g   (1 %)
- carbohydrates 53 g   (35%)
- added sugar   0 g   (0%)
- Fiber   7.9 g   (26%)

ingredients for 4 portions

- 1 orange
- ½ lemon
- 1 papaya
- 1 mango
- 200 g honeydew melon (1 piece)
- ½ pineapple
- 150 g physalis
- 150 g strawberries

preparation

Kitchen appliances

1 lemon squeezer, 1 knife, 1 work board

Preparation steps

1. Squeeze the orange and lemon halves. Peel the papaya, mango and half the pineapple.

2. Halve and core the papaya and chop the pulp. Remove the hard stalk from the pineapple; Cut the pulp into 1 cm cubes. Cut the mango pulp down at the core. Peel and core the melon. Roll both dice.

3. Clean and wash physalis. Wash and clean the strawberries and cut in halves or quarters. Mix the fruit with orange and lemon juice in a bowl and serve, for example, in small bowls

Cheese omelette with herbs

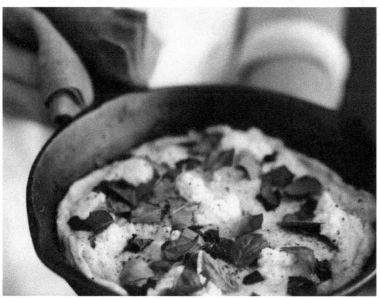

Preparation:

5 min

ready in 20 min

Calories:

335 kcal

Nutritional values

1 serving contains

(proportion of the daily requirement in percent)

- Calories335 kcal   (16%)
- protein 21 g   (21%)
- fat   27 g   (23%)
- carbohydrates 3 g   (2%)
- added sugar   0 g   (0%)
- Fiber   0.2 g   (1 %)

ingredients for 4 portions

- 3 stems chervil
- 3 stems basil
- 20 g parmesan
- 1 shallot
- 8th eggs
- 2 tbsp creme fraiche cheese
- 1 tbsp butter
- 150 g sheep cheese
- salt
- pepper

preparation

Kitchen appliances

1 ovenproof pan, 1 knife, 1 grater

Preparation steps

1. Wash the chervil and basil, shake dry and roughly chop. Grate the parmesan. Peel and finely dice shallot. Whisk the eggs with the crème fraîche, parmesan, chervil and half of the basil.

2. Melt the butter in an ovenproof pan, fry the shallot in it, pour in the eggs and crumble the feta over it. Bake in a preheated oven at 200 ° C (convection 180 ° C, gas: level 3) for about 10 minutes until golden brown.
3. Remove from the oven, season with salt, pepper and serve sprinkled with the remaining basil.

Millet tabbouleh with yogurt cream

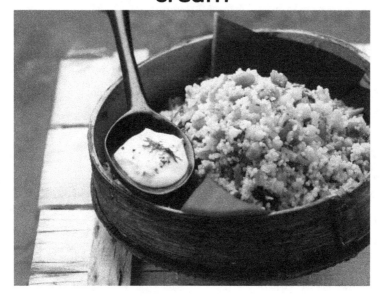

Preparation:

30 min

Calories:

597 kcal

Nutritional values

1 serving contains

(proportion of the daily requirement in percent)

- Calories597 kcal   (28%)
- protein 18 g   (18%)
- fat   23 g   (20%)
- carbohydrates 78 g   (52%)
- added sugar   0 g   (0%)
- Fiber   9.5 g   (32%)

ingredients for 4 portions

- 600 ml vegetable broth
- 375 g millet
- 30 g peanut kernel (unsalted; 2 tbsp)
- 1 red onion
- 1 red pepper
- 1 green pepper
- 1 yellow pepper
- 3 tbsp peanut oil
- 5 g coriander (0.25 bunch)
- 10 g parsley (0.5 bunch)
- 5 g mint (0.25 bunch)
- 300 g yogurt (3.5% fat)
- 100 g sour cream
- salt
- pepper
- 2 tbsp lemon juice

Preparation steps

1. Heat the broth in a saucepan. Rinse the millet in a sieve, add to the broth and let it soak over a low heat for 10–15 minutes. Then take it off the heat and loosen it up with a fork.
2. In the meantime, roast the peanuts in a pan without fat until they start to smell. Remove and set aside.
3. Peel onion and chop finely. Wash the peppers, cut in half, core and cut into fine cubes.
4. Heat 1 tablespoon of oil in a pan and sauté onions and peppers for 3–4 minutes. Take out and let cool down.
5. In the meantime, wash the herbs, shake them dry and roughly chop them separately. Mix coriander with yoghurt and sour cream and season with salt, pepper and 1 tablespoon of lemon juice.
6. Mix the parsley and mint with the millet, nuts, onions, paprika and the remaining oil. Season with salt, pepper and the remaining lemon juice. Spread the millet tabbouleh on 4 plates and serve with the yoghurt cream.

Shrimp salad with melon wedges

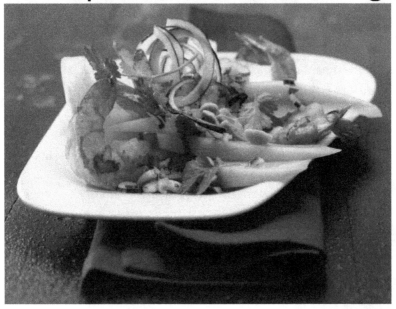

Preparation:

30 min

ready in 1 h 20 min

Calories:

190 kcal

Nutritional values

1 serving contains

(proportion of the daily requirement in percent)

- Calories 190 kcal   (9%)
- protein 16 g   (16%)
- fat   6 g   (5%)
- carbohydrates 16 g   (11%)
- added sugar   3 g   (12%)
- Fiber   3 g   (10%)

ingredients for 2 portions

- 125 g prawns (frozen, without shell)
- 70 g large red onions (1 large red onion)
- 1 red chilli pepper
- 1 lime
- 1 tbsp maple syrup
- salt
- 1 tsp rapeseed oil
- ½ melon (e.g., charentais)
- 15 g roasted, salted peanut kernel (1 tbsp)
- ½ fret coriander

preparation

Kitchen appliances

1 large plate, 1 work board, 1 small knife, 1 lemon squeezer, 1 tablespoon, 1 small bowl, 1 whisk, 1 small pan, 1 wooden spoon, 1 teaspoon, 1 large knife, 1 small pot with lid, 1 kitchen paper

Preparation steps

1. Thaw the prawns on a large plate according to the instructions on the packet.
2. In the meantime, peel the onion, cut off a few small rings and finely dice the rest of the onion.
3. Clean, wash, halve and core the chilli pepper and dice very finely.
4. Squeeze the lime. Mix 2 tablespoons of lime juice with maple syrup, 2 tablespoons of water, salt and chili cubes in a small bowl.
5. Score the defrosted shrimp along the back with a small knife and remove the black intestinal threads.
6. Rinse the prawns and pat dry with kitchen paper. Heat the oil in a small pan and fry the prawns for 3-4 minutes.
7. Add to the lime-chilli sauce while still warm with the onion cubes and let it steep for 10 minutes (marinate).
8. In the meantime, core the melon with a spoon, cut into 1 cm wide wedges and peel.
9. Roughly chop the peanuts with a large knife. Mix with the prawns.
10. Rinse the coriander, shake it dry, pluck the leaves off, roughly chop, also mix with the shrimp salad and season with salt. Arrange the salad with the melon wedges on plates, garnish with onion rings and serve.

Cheese and leek soup with tofu cubes

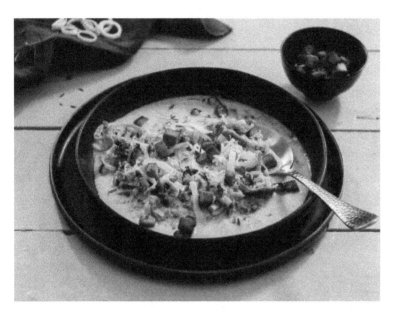

Preparation:

40 min

Calories:

433 kcal

Nutritional values

1 serving contains

(proportion of the daily requirement in percent)

- Calories 433 kcal   (21%)
- protein 21 g   (21%)
- fat   35 g   (30%)
- carbohydrates   8 g   (5%)
- added sugar   0 g   (0%)
- Fiber   4 g   (13%)

ingredients for 4 portions

- 200 g tofu
- 3 tbsp soy sauce
- 2 tbsp olive oil
- 1 tbsp vinegar
- 600 g leek
- 2 garlic cloves
- 4 branches thyme
- 2 tbsp coconut oil
- 100 g gouda cheese
- 150 g cream cheese
- 2 tsp mustard

preparation

Kitchen appliances

1 knife, 1 bowl, 1 saucepan, 1 grater, 1 coated pan

Preparation steps

1. Cut the tofu into cubes. Mix the soy sauce, oil and vinegar into a marinade and let the tofu cubes soak for about 30 minutes.
2. Clean, wash and cut the leek into fine rings, peel and finely chop the garlic. Wash the thyme, shake dry and pick off the leaves.
3. Melt 1 tbsp coconut oil in a saucepan and sauté the leek, garlic and half of the thyme over a medium heat for 1–2 minutes. Deglaze with 300 ml water and simmer over low heat for about 10 minutes.
4. Meanwhile grate Gouda. Stir the cream cheese and mustard into the soup.
5. Heat the rest of the coconut oil in a pan and fry the tofu cubes over a medium heat for about 5–7 minutes.
6. Stir the grated cheese into the soup, divide into 4 bowls and serve garnished with tofu cubes and the remaining thyme.

Zucchini soup with chanterelles and potatoes

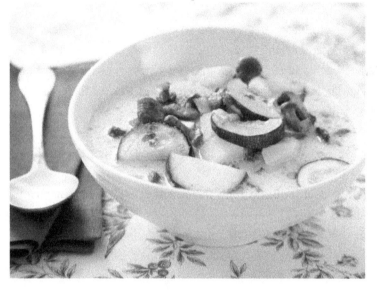

Preparation:

30 min

ready in 45 min

Calories:

265 kcal

Nutritional values

1 serving contains

(proportion of the daily requirement in percent)

- Calories 265 kcal   (13%)
- protein 6 g   (6%)
- fat   16 g   (14%)
- carbohydrates 23 g   (15%)
- added sugar   0 g   (0%)
- Fiber   3.8 g   (13%)

ingredients for 4 portions

- 500 g waxy potatoes
- 300 g zucchini
- 150 g fresh chanterelles
- 1 onion
- 1 clove of garlic
- 2 tbsp butter
- 750 ml of vegetable stock
- salt
- pepper
- 100 g sour cream
- nutmeg
- 2 tbsp olive oil
- 2 stems parsley

preparation

Kitchen appliances

1 saucepan, 1 hand blender, 1 coated pan

Preparation steps

1. Peel and wash the potatoes and cut into small, bite-sized pieces. Wash and clean zucchini as well, halve lengthways and cut into narrow slices. Clean and rub mushrooms.

2. Peel the onion and garlic, chop finely and sauté in a pan with melted butter until translucent. Add the potatoes and zucchini, sauté briefly and fill up with the stock. Salt, pepper and simmer over medium heat for about 10 minutes.

3. Remove half of the vegetables, set aside, puree the soup, stir in the sour cream and, if necessary, the stock and season with nutmeg.

4. Fry the mushrooms all around in a hot pan with 2 tablespoons of oil. Put the rest of the vegetables back into the soup and allow to warm up briefly. Wash parsley, shake dry and roughly chop. Divide the zucchini soup into bowls and serve sprinkled with parsley.

Chicken and zucchini salad with nuts

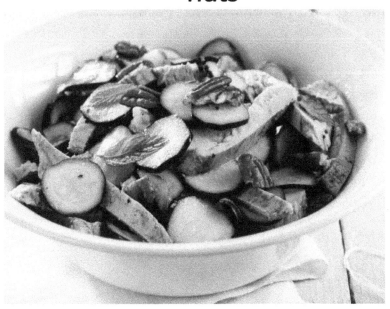

Preparation:

30 min

Calories:

399 kcal

Nutritional values

1 serving contains

(proportion of the daily requirement in percent)

- Calories399 kcal   (19%)
- protein 36 g   (37%)
- fat   26 g   (22%)

- carbohydrates 6 g (4%)
- added sugar 0 g (0%)
- Fiber 4.1 g (14%)

ingredients for 4 portions

- 3 zucchinis
- 500 g chicken breast fillet
- salt
- pepper
- 4 tbsp olive oil
- ½ fret mint
- ½ lemon
- 80 g pecans

preparation

Kitchen appliances

1 knife, 1 work board, 1 pan, 1 lemon squeezer

Preparation steps

1. Wash and clean the zucchini and cut into thin slices. Rinse the chicken fillet under cold water, pat dry, season with salt and pepper.
2. Heat 2 tablespoons of oil in a pan. Fry the chicken in it over medium heat for about 10 minutes until golden brown. Reduce the heat and let the chicken breast fillets cook.
3. Heat the remaining oil in another pan. Sauté zucchini slices in it over medium heat for about 4 minutes.
4. Wash the mint, shake dry and pluck the leaves. Squeeze half lemons.
5. Remove the chicken from the pan, drain on kitchen paper and cut into thin slices. Roughly chop the nuts and mix with the zucchini, chicken, mint and lemon juice. Season with salt and pepper and arrange in bowls.

Filled omelette

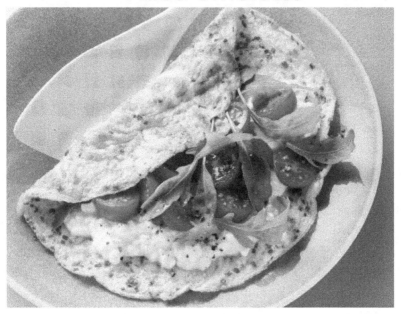

Preparation:

20 min

ready in 35 min

Calories:

250 kcal

Nutritional values

1 serving contains

(proportion of the daily requirement in percent)

- Calories250 kcal   (12%)
- protein 19 g   (19%)
- fat   17 g   (15%)

- carbohydrates 5 g (3%)
- added sugar 0 g (0%)
- Fiber 1.3 g (4%)

ingredients for 4 portions

- 40 g rocket (1 handful)
- 300 g cherry tomatoes
- 10 g chives (0.5 bunch)
- 8th eggs
- 4 tbsp carbonated mineral water
- salt
- pepper
- nutmeg
- 4 tsp sunflower oil
- 150 g grained cream cheese

Preparation steps

1. Wash the rocket and spin dry. Wash tomatoes and cut in half. Wash the chives, shake dry and cut into rolls.
2. Whisk eggs with water and chives and season with salt, pepper and freshly grated nutmeg.
3. Heat 1 teaspoon sunflower oil in a coated pan and add 1/4 of the egg milk. Fry for 2 minutes over medium heat, turn and finish cooking in another 2 minutes. Take out and keep warm in the preheated oven at 80 ° C (convection 60 ° C; gas: lowest setting). Bake 3 more omelets in this way.
4. Place omelets on 4 plates and fill with cream cheese, tomatoes and rocket. Season with salt and pepper and whip in.

Buckwheat pancakes with blueberries

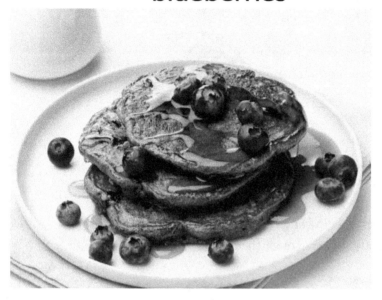

Preparation:

20 min

ready in 50 min

Calories:

399 kcal

Nutritional values

1 serving contains

(proportion of the daily requirement in percent)

- Calories 399 kcal (19%)
- protein 8.5 g (9%)
- fat 7.5 g (6%)
- carbohydrates 75.5 g (50%)

- added sugar   11 g   (44%)
- Fiber   7.4 g   (25%)

ingredients for 4 portions

- 300 ml oat drink (oat milk)
- 150 g coconut yogurt
- 3 tbsp rice syrup
- 1 pinch
- salt
- 250 g buckwheat flour
- 2 tsp baking powder
- 300 g blueberries (fresh or frozen)
- 2 tbsp rapeseed oil
- 2 tbsp maple syrup

preparation

Kitchen appliances

1 bowl, 1 pan, 1 whisk

Preparation steps

1. Whisk the oat drink with coconut yoghurt, rice syrup and a pinch of salt. Mix the flour with baking powder and add to the yogurt mixture while stirring. Mix everything into a smooth dough and let rest for about 30 minutes.
2. In the meantime, thaw the blueberries or wash and drain them.
3. Heat oil in a pan. Add 2 tablespoons of batter to each pancake, sprinkle with a few blueberries and fry on both sides over medium heat for 1–2 minutes each until golden brown. In this way, use up all of the batter.
4. Stack the pancakes on 4 plates, sprinkle with the remaining berries and drizzle with maple syrup

Grilled potato and bacon skewers

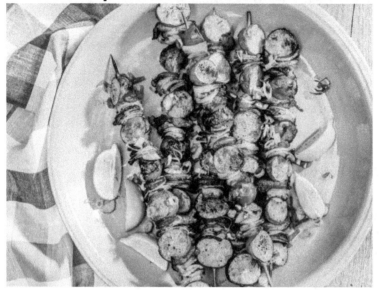

Preparation:

20 min

ready in 35 min

Calories:

705 kcal

Nutritional values

1 serving contains

(proportion of the daily requirement in percent)

- Calories 705 kcal (34%)
- protein 12 g (12%)
- fat 45 g (39%)
- carbohydrates 61 g (41%)
- added sugar 0 g (0%)

- Fiber   5.2 g   (17%)

ingredients for 4 portions

- 1 ½ kg cooked, small new potatoes
- 2 onions
- 150 g turkey bacon, sliced
- 4 tbsp rapeseed oil
- salt
- pepper from the mill
- 2 spring onions
- 2 tbsp lemon juice

preparation

Kitchen appliances

1 knife, 1 work board, 8 wooden skewers, 1 bowl, 1 grill

Preparation steps

1. Halve the potatoes. Peel and quarter the onions and cut into individual slices. Alternate with the potatoes and the folded bacon slices on long wooden skewers (preferably soaked beforehand). Brush with oil, season with salt and pepper and cook on the hot grill for about 15 minutes, turning regularly.
2. Wash and clean the spring onions and cut into rings. Mix with the remaining oil, lemon juice, salt and pepper.
3. Remove the skewers from the grill and serve drizzled with the spring onion vinaigrette.

Grilled zucchini flowers with pecorino

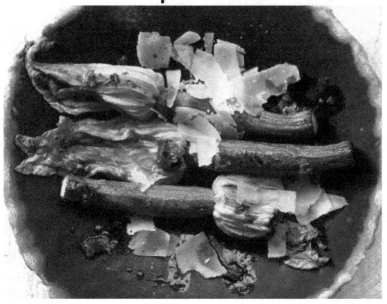

Preparation:

20 min

ready in 35 min

Calories:

146 kcal

Nutritional values

1 serving contains

(proportion of the daily requirement in percent)

- Calories146 kcal   (7%)
- protein 4 g   (4%)
- fat   14 g   (12%)
- carbohydrates 1 g   (1 %)
- added sugar   0 g   (0%)
- Fiber   0.4 g   (1 %)

ingredients for 4 portions

- 8th zucchini flowers
- 2 sun-dried tomatoes
- 3 stems oregano
- 1 lime
- 4 tbsp olive oil
- 50 g pecorino
- salt
- pepper

preparation

Kitchen appliances

1 small bowl, 1 work board, 1 small knife, 1 tablespoon, 1 peeler, 1 spatula, 1 grill pan, 1 lemon squeezer

Preparation steps

1. Remove the pointed outer sepals around the base of the stalk.
2. Carefully open the flowers, remove the pistils and then cut off the lower ends of the flowers.
3. Finely chop the dried tomatoes. Wash the oregano, shake dry, pluck the leaves, chop finely and place in a bowl with the squeezed lime juice.
4. Stir in olive oil.
5. Finely slice the pecorino cheese with the peeler.
6. Heat a grill pan or grill. Grill the flowers in it over medium heat for 4–5 minutes, then place on a plate, season with salt and pepper and immediately drizzle with the marinade. Pour cheese over it and let it steep for 15 minutes.

Mashed potatoes with pointed cabbage and horseradish

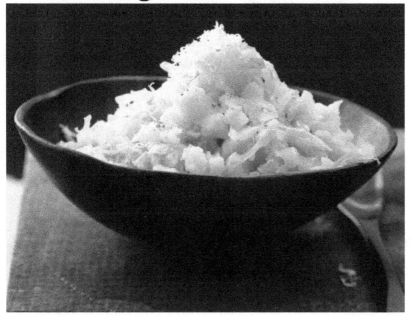

Preparation:

45 min

Calories:

257 kcal

Nutritional values

1 serving contains

(proportion of the daily requirement in percent)

- Calories257 kcal   (12%)
- protein 10 g   (10%)

- fat   6 g   (5%)
- carbohydrates 36 g   (24%)
- added sugar   0 g   (0%)
- Fiber   9.5 g   (32%)

ingredients for 2 portions

- 500 g floury potatoes
- salt
- 300 g small pointed cabbage (0.5 small pointed cabbage)
- 2 small onions
- 2 tbsp rapeseed oil
- 100 ml milk (1.5% fat)
- pepper
- 1 piece
- horseradish (approx. 3 cm long)

preparation

Kitchen appliances

2 pots, 1 bowl, 1 measuring cup, 1 work board, 1 large knife, 1 small knife, 1 tablespoon, 1 wooden spoon, 1 peeler, 1 fine grater, 1 sieve, 1 potato masher, 1 lid

Preparation steps

1. Wash, peel and dice the potatoes. Bring to the boil in salted water and cook covered for 20 minutes.
2. While the potatoes are boiling, clean the pointed cabbage, remove the stalk in a wedge shape if necessary, cut the cabbage into very fine strips across the leaf veins.
3. Peel the onions and finely dice them.
4. Heat oil in a pan. Add onion cubes and sauté for 2 minutes over medium heat until translucent. Add the pointed cabbage and cook for 3 minutes while stirring.
5. Pour in milk and bring to the boil once. Season with salt and pepper.
6. Drain the potatoes and let them evaporate briefly. Coarsely mash the potatoes with a potato masher.
7. Add the potatoes to the pointed cabbage and mix in.
8. Peel the horseradish, grate it finely and mix it with the mashed potatoes. Season everything with salt and pepper and serve immediately.

Keto bowl with konjac noodles and peanut sauce

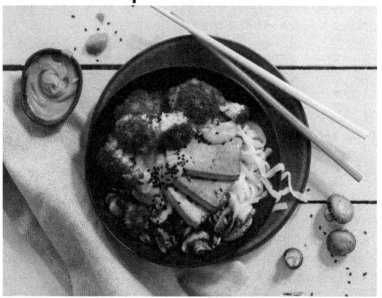

Preparation:

30 min

ready in 50 min

Calories:

621 kcal

Nutritional values

1 serving contains

(proportion of the daily requirement in percent)

- Calories 621 kcal   (30%)
- protein 42 g   (43%)
- fat   44 g   (38%)

- carbohydrates 10 g (7%)
- added sugar 0 g (0%)
- Fiber 13 g (43%)

ingredients for 2 portions

- 300 g tofu
- 1 clove of garlic
- 20th ginger
- 35 ml soy sauce
- 10 ml rice vinegar
- 1 shallot
- 200 g mushrooms
- 200 g broccoli
- 3 tbsp sesame oil
- salt
- pepper from the grinder
- 50 g peanut butter
- 50 ml coconut milk
- 400 g konjac noodles
- 1 tsp black sesame

Preparation

Kitchen appliances

1 knife, 1 coated pan, 1 saucepan

Preparation steps

1. Cut the tofu into 8 slices. Peel the garlic and ginger and cut very finely. Mix the garlic, ginger, 30 ml soy sauce and rice vinegar. Marinate the tofu with it and let it steep for 20 minutes.

2. In the meantime, peel the shallot and cut into small pieces. Clean mushrooms. Wash broccoli and cut into florets. Heat 1 tablespoon of oil in a pan and fry the shallot and mushrooms over medium heat for 5–8 minutes. Season with salt and pepper. Cook the broccoli in salted boiling water for 3 minutes. Take out and drain.

3. For the peanut sauce, put peanut butter and coconut milk in a saucepan and heat. Season with cayenne pepper and the rest of the soy sauce.

4. Take the mushrooms out of the pan. Heat the rest of the oil in the pan and fry the tofu on both sides for 4 minutes on a medium heat.

5. Rinse konjak spaghetti thoroughly and cook in salted boiling water for 2 minutes. Pouring off. Serve the mushroom mix with broccoli, konjac spaghetti and tofu. Drizzle with the peanut sauce. Serve the keto bowl sprinkled with sesame seeds.

Keto lasagna

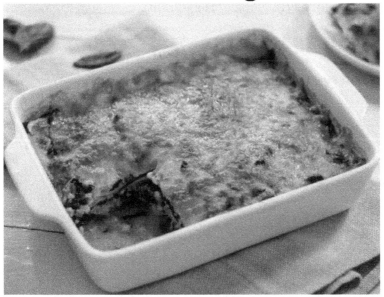

Preparation:

30 min

ready in 55 min

Calories:

541 kcal

Nutritional values

1 serving contains

(proportion of the daily requirement in percent)

- Calories 541 kcal   (26%)
- protein 35 g   (36%)
- fat   40 g   (34%)
- carbohydrates 9 g   (6%)
- added sugar   0 g   (0%)
- Fiber   119 g   (397%)

ingredients for 4 portions

- 150 g soy cutlets
- 300 g spinach
- 1 shallot
- 2 tbsp olive oil
- 1 tbsp tomato paste
- 200 ml vegetable broth
- salt
- pepper
- 5 g yeast flakes
- 200 g whipped cream
- 100 g sour cream
- 1 pinch nutmeg
- 1 tsp guar gum
- 400 g zucchini
- 150 g mozzarella

preparation

Kitchen appliances

1 bowl, 1 coated pan, 1 small sieve, 1 peeler

Preparation steps

1. Soak the soy in hot water for 10–15 minutes according to the instructions on the package, then pour off any remaining liquid. Clean and wash the spinach and spin dry. Peel and finely chop shallot.
2. Heat the olive oil in a large pan, fry the shallot and soy in it over medium heat for about 5–7 minutes, add the tomato paste and fry briefly, then add the spinach, deglaze with the vegetable stock, bring to the boil and season with salt, pepper and yeast flakes.
3. Mix the whipped cream with sour cream, salt, pepper and nutmeg. Put guar gum through a sieve and gradually stir in until it has a slightly viscous consistency.
4. Clean and wash the zucchini and cut lengthways into thin slices, the easiest way to do this is with a vegetable peeler. Drain the mozzarella and cut into small cubes.
5. Alternate in a baking dish, layer soy spinach with creamy cream and zucchini plates like a classic lasagne, top with creamy cream and sprinkle with mozzarella for about 25 minutes in a preheated oven at 180 ° C (convection 160 ° C, gas: level 2-3) bake, switch to the oven's grill function for the last 3 minutes.

CONCLUSION

Eating gluten-free does not harm adults, but the bottom line is that it makes little sense as a slimming diet. Suitable for: people with celiac disease or in consultation with a doctor. If you want to lose weight, you should focus on the entire diet and not on a single active ingredient.

A gluten-free diet is currently the only therapy that guarantees optimal health for people with celiac disease. The solution for celiac disease is to permanently avoid all foods that are made from gluten-containing grains or contain gluten. Even the smallest traces of gluten can cause histological damage, so special care is required. People with celiac disease must therefore pay particular attention to the selection of their food.

HEALTY

DAIRY- FREE

RECIPES

simple and Delicious Recipes for Cooking with Whole Foods on a Restrictive Diet

Jhon newman

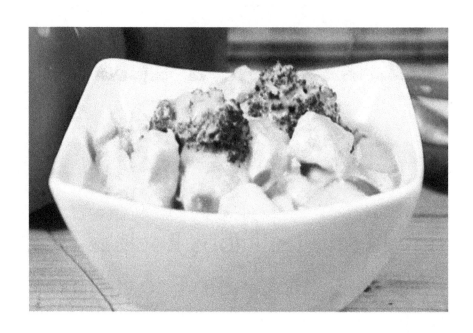

All rights reserved.

Disclaimer

INTRODUCTION

DAIRY-FREE DIET

The cow 's milk is a complete food, rich in nutrients and especially needed during the growing season but in recent years, numerous researches suggests that milk also has its drawbacks and that not everything in it are benefits health. A dairy-free diet implies excluding milk of animal origin and all its derivatives, which are many: butter, cheeses, yogurts, cream, ice cream ... not counting all the processed products that may contain it.

Some people have different degrees of allergy to milk proteins, mainly casein, and also intolerance to its sugars, with Dairy in the first place. In these cases, eliminating dairy is essential to avoid adverse reactions that can range from digestive problems such as nausea or diarrhea, to complications in the respiratory system.

The benefits of a dairy-free diet

1. Improved digestion

As we have said, cow 's milk is a food of great nutritional value but we must take into account its high fat content, 3.7%, which is mostly saturated fat. It should also be noted its richness in sugars, mainly Dairy, a carbohydrate that, in general, is difficult to digest and is practically impossible for people who lack the enzymes responsible for breaking it down, so they develop intolerance. For all this, eliminating dairy in many cases means significantly lighter digestions.

2. Avoid reflux and other gastrointestinal problems

In relation to the above, some studies confirm that more than 70% of the world population has some degree of Dairy intolerance (many do not know it). Common ailments such as a simple stomach ache, cramps or cramps, nausea or excessive gas can be caused by excessive consumption of dairy products. Milk is not the best alidade of gastritis or reflux, since, due to its "rebound" effect, it increases acidity.

3. Promotes the good condition of the respiratory tract

It is another benefit that, according to some experts, produces the suppression of dairy. The reason is that its continued presence in the diet favors the appearance and increase of mucus, complicating respiratory ailments such as asthma.

4. Lower risk of developing some types of cancer

Without being alarmist, because this statement is not confirmed, certain investigations link the continued intake of cow's milk and derivatives with the appearance of prostate and ovarian cancer. Milk is also believed to contribute to irritable bowel syndrome.

5. Improvement of skin conditions

Due to the hormonal treatments (steroids and anabolic) to which, on many occasions, cattle are subjected, the elimination of dairy products can contribute to the improvement of the condition of the skin in general, making problems such as acne.

6. Less cholesterol

The numbers speak for themselves. Whole cow's milk has 14% cholesterol. It is clear that people who have a high level of bad cholesterol in their blood should do without it or at least limit their consumption.

As you can see, milk is not in all cases as healthy a food as has always been believed. Perhaps for this reason, many people have eliminated it from their diet, either for health or personal conviction. In these cases, we must take into account that we must substitute dairy products of animal origin for other foods that provide us with the essential nutrients it contains, that is, its essential vitamins and minerals such as calcium, phosphorus, vitamin D or those of group B (B2 and B12). The vegetable milk, soy, almond, walnut and some foods such as broccoli, kale or watercress are especially recommended if you removed milk of your diet.

Who Needs Dairy-Free Food?

Dairy-free foods contain milk sugar that has already been broken down. Since your body lacks the enzyme lactase, which normally breaks down milk sugar, such foods are easier to digest for people with lactose intolerance. People without this intolerance do not gain any added value from consuming Dairy-free foods, even if this is often assumed.

Dairy-Free Food List

With the exception of milk, dairy products and cheese, foods are naturally lactose-free. The safest diet is therefore a diet in which as much fresh and unprocessed food as possible is selected and milk and fresh dairy products are replaced with Dairy-free alternatives.

The following foods do not contain lactose:

- Fruit juices, mineral water, tea, coffee
- fruit
- vegetables
- Nuts and almonds
- Legumes, tofu
- Potatoes, pasta, rice
- Cereals, cereal flakes
- Dairy-free milk and dairy products
- Hard and semi-hard cheese
- Chicken egg, boiled egg, fried egg
- Meat and meat products such as cold roasts, roast beef, corned beef
- Sausage (ask about ingredients)
- fish and seafood
- natural vegetable oils, Dairy-free margarine, clarified butter, (butter)
- Herbs, spices
- Honey, jam
- Sugar beet syrup, molasses, apple cabbage, pear cabbage
- Fruit gums without yogurt

DAIRY-FREE RECIPES

LEMON CHICKEN WITH BROCCOLI

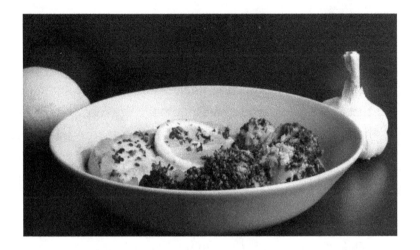

Ingredients for 4 servings

- 2 chicken breast fillets (approx. 500 g)
- 1 KG frozen broccoli
- 1 onion (medium)
- 4 cloves of garlic
- 1 can of coconut milk (400 ml)
- 2 tsp vegetable broth
- 2 teaspoons of poultry broth
- 1 lemon
- 2 tbsp parsley (fresh)
- 2 teaspoons of cornstarch

- 1 tbsp coconut oil
- ½ teaspoon salt
- 1 teaspoon black pepper

Preparation time: 10 mins

preparation

1. Dab the chicken breast fillets with a paper towel and cut in half. Peel onion and chop finely. Peel the garlic and pass it through a garlic press. Wash lemon. Squeeze the juice of half a lemon. Cut the other half of the lemon into slices. Wash and roughly chop the parsley.
2. Put the broccoli in a saucepan with a little water and the vegetable stock. Bring to the boil and remove from heat as soon as the broccoli is cooked firm to the bite.
3. While the broccoli is steaming, heat coconut oil in a non-stick frying pan over a medium to high flame. Fry the chicken breast fillets for approx. 5 minutes on each side, until they are golden brown. Place the chicken on a plate and set aside.
4. Reduce the heat to medium heat. Add onions, garlic, salt and pepper and fry for about 1 minute, stirring occasionally.
5. Stir in coconut milk, broth and lemon juice and bring to a boil. Mix 2 teaspoons of cornstarch and 2 teaspoons of water in a glass with a fork and stir into the sauce. Return the chicken to the pan and simmer until the sauce has thickened slightly. Garnish the lemon chicken with parsley and lemon wedges. Then serve with the broccoli.

Nutritional information / 1 serving

- Calories 486 Kcal
- carbohydrates 16 g
- Proteins 43 g
- Fat 26 g

CHICKEN CURRY WITH COCONUT MILK

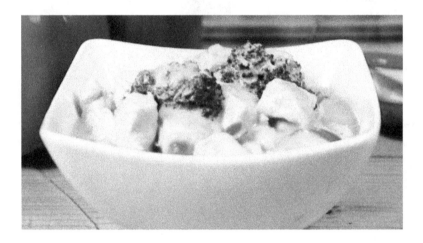

Ingredients for 3 servings

- 500 g chicken breast fillet
- 200 g frozen broccoli
- 1 bell pepper (red)
- 1 onion
- 1 can of coconut milk (400ml)
- 3 cloves of garlic
- 1 tbsp curry powder
- 1/2 teaspoon red curry paste
- ¼ tsp chili powder
- 1 teaspoon turmeric
- 1 teaspoon honey
- 1 tbsp rapeseed oil

- 1 pinch of salt

Preparation time: 25 mins

preparation

1. Cut the chicken into 2 cm cubes. Peel and dice the onion. Wash and core the peppers and cut into small pieces. Peel the garlic and pass it through a garlic press.
2. Heat the rapeseed oil in a large pan over medium heat. Add the chicken and sauté until golden brown on all sides. Add broccoli, onion and paprika and fry for 5 minutes, stirring occasionally.
3. Add coconut milk, curry powder, red curry paste, chili powder, turmeric, honey, garlic and salt and stir vigorously. Reduce the heat to low heat and let the chicken curry steep for 5 minutes with the lid closed. Stir occasionally. Then serve.

Nutritional information / 1 serving

- Calories 518 Kcal
- carbohydrates 22 g
- Proteins 44 g
- Fat 32 g

CARROT AND GINGER SOUP

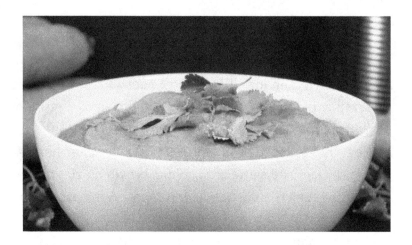

Ingredients for 4 servings

- ingredients
- 1 KG carrots
- 1 can of coconut milk (400 ml)
- 50 ml orange juice
- 40 g ginger
- 1 chilli pepper (small)
- 3 tsp vegetable broth
- 1 teaspoon pepper
- ½ teaspoon salt
- ½ teaspoon paprika powder (noble sweet)
- ½ teaspoon paprika powder (hot pink)
- 1 strand of coriander (to garnish)

Preparation time: 30 mins

preparation

1. Peel the carrots and cut into slices. Peel and chop the ginger. Remove the seeds from the chilli and then cut the chilli pepper into small pieces.
2. Put the carrots in a large saucepan with coconut milk, orange juice, ginger, chilli pepper, vegetable stock, pepper, salt and paprika powder. Simmer under high to medium heat for about 15 minutes with the lid on.
3. Puree everything with a hand blender to make a soup. Garnish with coriander. Then serve.

Nutritional information / 1 serving

- Calories 321 Kcal
- carbohydrates 31 g
- Proteins 5 g
- Fat 23 g

PEA SOUP WITH FROZEN PEAS

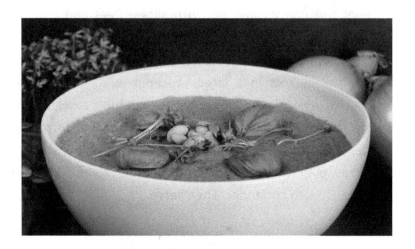

Ingredients for 4 servings

- 1 KG frozen peas
- 1 green onion
- 1 teaspoon ginger (fresh)
- 400 ml coconut milk
- 100 ml almond milk
- 2 ½ teaspoons vegetable stock
- 1 ½ tsp nutmeg
- 1 ½ tsp pepper
- ½ teaspoon salt
- 1 teaspoon coriander
- 2 cloves of garlic
- 30 g pine nuts

- 1 tbsp coconut oil
- Basil (to garnish)
- Cress (to garnish)

Preparation time: 25 mins

preparation

1. Peel and dice the onion. Peel the ginger and garlic and cut into small pieces.
2. Heat coconut oil in a large saucepan over high heat and briefly fry the onions with the ginger and garlic until the onions are translucent.
3. Add coconut milk, almond milk, vegetable stock and frozen peas and reduce everything over medium heat for 10 minutes, stirring occasionally. At the same time, roast the pine nuts in a coated pan until golden brown, stirring constantly.
4. Add nutmeg, coriander, pepper and salt. Puree everything into a pea soup. Garnish with pine nuts, basil and cress as desired. Then serve.

Nutritional information / 1 serving

- Calories 490 Kcal
- carbohydrates 46 g
- Fiber 15 g
- Proteins 17 g
- Fat 28 g

CREAMY CHICKEN KORMA WITH BROCCOLI

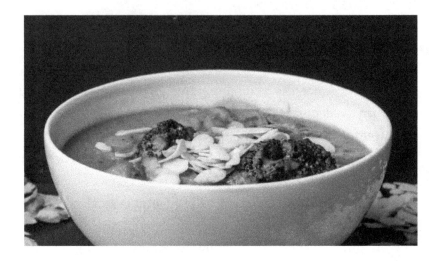

Ingredients for 3 servings

- 400 g chicken breast fillet
- 400 g broccoli
- 2 onions
- 1 teaspoon ginger
- 3 cloves of garlic
- 400 ml of pureed tomatoes
- 400 ml coconut milk
- 2 teaspoons of ground cumin
- 1 teaspoon coriander
- 1 teaspoon turmeric
- 1 teaspoon red chili paste

- ½ teaspoon cinnamon
- ½ teaspoon nutmeg
- ½ teaspoon salt
- ½ teaspoon black pepper
- 1 tbsp coconut oil
- Almond flakes (for garnish)

Preparation time: 30 mins

preparation

1. Cut the chicken breast fillets into small pieces (approx. 2.5 cm). Wash broccoli and separate broccoli florets. Peel and dice the onions. Peel and chop the ginger. Peel the garlic cloves and pass them through a garlic press.
2. Heat ½ tbsp coconut oil in a large, non-stick pan over medium heat and fry the chicken for about 5 minutes on all sides. Turn occasionally, then take the chicken out of the pan and pour off any liquid.
3. Add ½ tbsp coconut oil to the pan and fry the ginger with garlic over medium heat for a minute. Then add the onions and fry for 3 minutes, stirring frequently, until the onions are translucent.
4. Add the tomatoes, coconut milk and broccoli. Return the chicken to the pan. Season with ground cumin, coriander, turmeric, red chilli paste, cinnamon, nutmeg, salt and black pepper. Mix vigorously, then simmer for about 10 minutes with the lid closed. Garnish with toasted almond flakes Then serve.

Nutritional information / 1 serving

- Calories 604 Kcal
- carbohydrates 32 g
- Fiber 12 g
- Proteins 41 g
- Fat 37 g

QUICK BROWNIE PORRIDGE

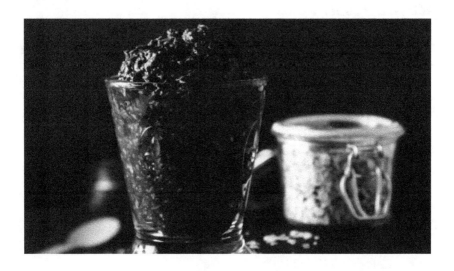

Ingredients for 2 servings

- 1 cup (250ml) almond or coconut milk
- 1 cup (250ml) oats
- 1/2 cup (125 ml) natural Greek yogurt, low in fat
- 1-2 tbsp cocoa powder
- 2-3 tbsp honey
- 30g chocolate protein (or extra oatmeal)
- Dark chocolate pieces

Preparation time: 5 mins

preparation

1. Mix the dry ingredients together first, then mix them in with everything else.
2. Divide the porridge into 2 bowls and serve immediately or let it set overnight in the refrigerator. Just try out both variants and see which one you like best.

Nutritional information / 1 serving

- Calories 320 Kcal
- carbohydrates 44 g
- Fiber 6 g
- Proteins 21 g
- Fat 6 g

ROASTED "CAPRESE" CHICKEN BREAST WITH TOMATOES, BASIL AND MOZZARELLA

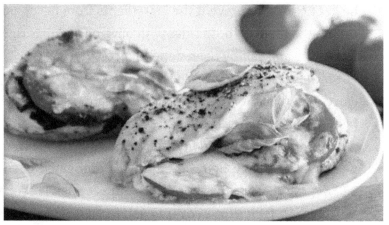

Ingredients for 4 servings

- 800g (4 medium-sized pieces) chicken breast
- 200g fresh mozzarella
- a handful of fresh basil
- 2 tomatoes
- ground black pepper (to taste)
- Salt (to taste)
- Garlic powder (to taste)
- Balsamic vinegar (optional)
- 1-2 tbsp olive oil

Preparation time: 35 mins

preparation

1. Cut the chicken breast on one side. The other side should be kept closed to prevent the ingredients from falling out.
2. Drizzle the meat on both sides with olive oil and massage in the spices and salt by hand depending on your taste.
3. Cut tomatoes and mozzarella into thin slices.
4. Place a few slices of mozzarella and tomatoes in each piece of meat. Also add basil leaves.
5. Place the stuffed chicken breasts in a baking dish.
6. Bake the meat (can be covered) in the preheated oven at 220 degrees Celsius for about 20 minutes until it is cooked. After baking, let it sit in a covered pan for at least 5 minutes.
7. Finally, you can add balsamic vinegar and serve it with your favorite side dish.

Nutritional information / 1 serving

- Calories 403 Kcal
- carbohydrates 3 g
- Fiber   1 g
- Proteins 55 g
- Fat 16 g

SIMPLE GRILLED CHICKEN BREAST WITH BASIL AND STRAWBERRIES

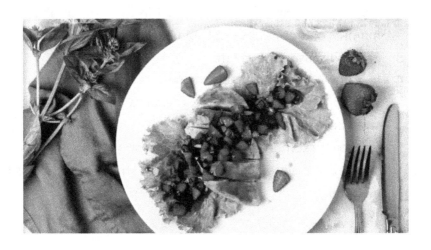

Ingredients for 2 servings

- 300g chicken breast
- 2 teaspoons coconut oil (or olive oil)
- 2 cloves of garlic
- 1/2 teaspoon sea salt
- 1/2 teaspoon ground black pepper
- 300g strawberries
- a handful of basil leaves
- Spinach / lettuce leaves
- 3 tbsp balsamic vinegar

Preparation time: 15 mins

preparation

1. Heat 1 teaspoon of oil in a grill pan and lightly fry the pressed garlic cloves.
2. Fry the thinly sliced chicken breast in the pan for about 3 minutes on both sides until golden brown.
3. Salt and season the meat.
4. In a bowl, mix a teaspoon of melted coconut oil, balsamic vinegar, finely chopped basil, and washed and sliced strawberries.
5. Grilled chicken breast can be served on spinach or lettuce leaves and covered with the prepared strawberry and basil mixture.

Nutritional information / 1 serving

- Calories 285 Kcal
- carbohydrates 7 g
- Fiber 4 g
- Proteins 40 g
- Fat 7 g

SIMPLY BAKED CHICKEN NUGGETS IN A YOGURT CRUST

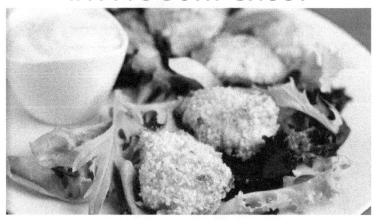

Ingredients for 4 servings

- 400g chicken breast
- 200g whole meal breading flour (or corn crumbs / ground almonds)
- 200g natural yogurt
- 1 teaspoon salt
- 1 tbsp garlic powder
- a pinch of ground black pepper
- 2 tbsp grated Parmesan cheese (optional)

for the sauce:

- 250g natural yogurt
- 2 tbsp mustard
- 1 tbsp honey

Preparation time: 50 mins

preparation

1. Wash the chicken breast and cut into smaller pieces.
2. Mix the yogurt with salt, pepper and grated parmesan in a bowl.
3. Spread the yogurt mixture on the chicken pieces, then coat them with whole wheat breading, corn crumbs, or ground almonds.
4. Place the breaded pieces on a baking sheet lined with baking paper and bake for 30-35 minutes at 190 ° C until crispy. You can turn them over in the middle of the baking process.
5. Prepare the sauce by mixing together yogurt, mustard, and honey. You can let them rest in the refrigerator before serving.
6. As a side dish, you can choose either a salad, potatoes or rice.

Nutritional information / 1 serving

- Calories 397 Kcal
- carbohydrates 46 g
- Fiber 3 g
- Proteins 36 g
- Fat 6 g

SIMPLE CELERY AND BROCCOLI SOUP

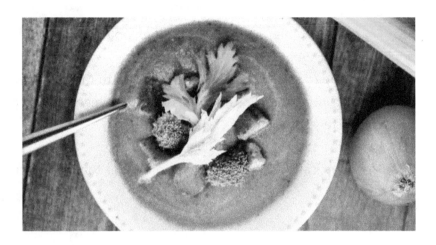

Ingredients for 4 servings

- 4 celery stalks
- 1 large broccoli
- 1 ½ liters of vegetable stock
- 1 tbsp olive oil
- 1 onion
- 3 cloves of garlic
- 1 teaspoon sea salt
- ½ teaspoon ground black pepper
- coriander
- thyme

Preparation time: 25 mins

preparation

1. Lightly fry the finely chopped onion in oil in a saucepan.
2. Add the washed and finely chopped celery stalks and broccoli.
3. Fry the vegetables for a while and then pour the vegetable stock over them.
4. Add pepper, salt and crushed garlic cloves to the soup and cook covered for 15-20 minutes until the vegetables are completely soft.
5. Puree the soup with a hand blender.
6. The soup can be served with whole meal toast cut into cubes.

Nutritional information / 1 serving

- Calories 72 Kcal
- carbohydrates 4 g
- Fiber   5 g
- Proteins 4 g
- Fat 4 g

SIMPLE HOKKAIDO PUMPKIN SOUP

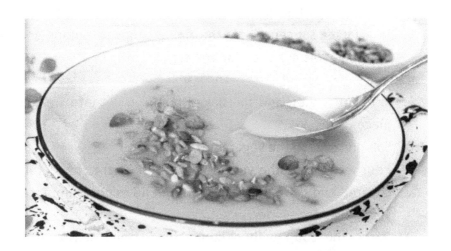

Ingredients for 6 servings

- 800g Hokkaido pumpkin (after peeling)
- 200g carrots
- 2 parsley
- 1 large onion
- 3 cloves of garlic
- 1 tbsp oil / butter
- sea-salt
- ground black pepper
- Curry powder / turmeric
- Pumpkin and sunflower seeds (optional)

Preparation time: 50 mins

preparation

1. Halve the pumpkin and bake at 200 degrees for 15-20 minutes until tender.
2. Let cool after baking, then peel and cut out the stones.
3. In a larger saucepan, fry the finely chopped onions and crushed garlic in hot oil (or butter).
4. Add the chopped carrots and parsley.
5. Fry lightly, then add the baked pumpkin cut into smaller pieces.
6. Salt and season the vegetables to taste.
7. Pour water over the vegetables until they are completely covered and cook the soup for about 15 minutes until the vegetables are tender.
8. Puree the soup with a hand blender and season it if necessary.
9. The soup can be served sprinkled with dry, roasted pumpkin seeds or other seeds (highly recommended! :)).

Nutritional information / 1 serving

- Calories 57 Kcal
- carbohydrates 8 g
- Fiber 3 g
- Proteins 2 g
- Fat 2 g

ZUCCHINI SPAGHETTI (ZOODLES) WITH CREAMY AVOCADO SAUCE AND SALMON

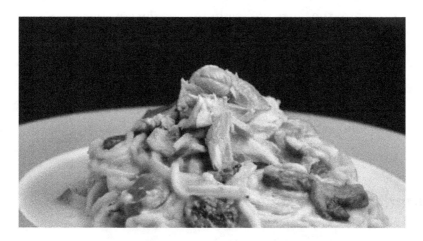

Ingredients for 2 servings

- 300 g salmon (possibly chicken breast)
- 1 zucchini
- 1 avocado
- 200 g mushrooms
- 3 tbsp yogurt
- Juice from 1 lime
- 1/3 onion
- 1 clove of garlic
- parsley
- 1/2 teaspoon sea salt
- 1/2 teaspoon pepper

Preparation time: 15 mins

preparation

1. Grill the salmon together with the mushrooms until golden brown.
2. Grate the zucchini with the peeler or the grater into spaghetti and place in a bowl.
3. Puree the avocado, yogurt, lime juice, garlic, onion, pepper, salt and a little parsley in a blender.
4. Mix the finished sauce with the zucchini spaghetti and the salmon champion mixture and serve warm.

Nutritional information / 1 serving

- Calories 375 Kcal
- carbohydrates 8 g
- Fiber   7 g
- Proteins 35 g
- Fat 21 g

HEALTHY BAKED CARROT BALLS

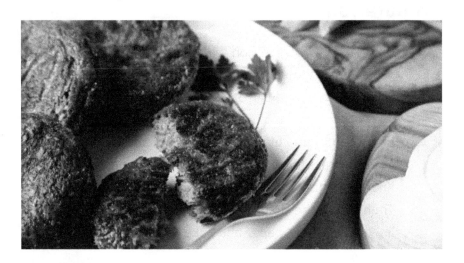

Ingredients for 8 servings

- 500 g carrots
- 1 onion
- 2 eggs
- 2 cloves of garlic
- 5 tbsp whole meal / oat / chickpea flour
- 1 teaspoon sea salt
- 1 teaspoon marjoram
- ½ teaspoon ground pepper

Preparation time: 45 mins

preparation

1. Grate the carrots, season with salt and then steam with a little water (about 5 minutes).
2. Sieve the steamed carrots and squeeze out the remaining water.
3. Peel the onion, cut into small pieces and knead with the carrots, pressed garlic, spices, eggs and the chosen flour.
4. Knead the dough well and let it stand for 10 minutes.
5. Then shape the dough into balls, place on a baking sheet lined with baking paper and bake

Nutritional information / 1 serving

- Calories 52 Kcal
- carbohydrates 6 g
- Fiber 2 g
- Proteins 3 g
- Fat 1 g

HEALTHY EGG MUFFINS WITH TUNA

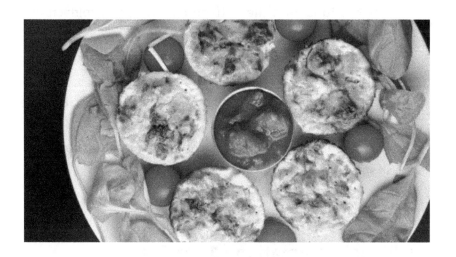

Ingredients for 6 servings

- 120 g of tuna in its own juice
- 2 eggs
- 4 tbsp cottage cheese
- 1 handful of spinach (fresh)
- 1 pinch of ground pepper
- 1 pinch of sea salt
- grated cheese (optional)

Preparation time: 40 mins

preparation

1. Mix the tuna with the cottage cheese, eggs, spinach and pepper in a bowl.
2. For an even more delicious taste, you can also use some grated cheese.
3. Fill the resulting dough into muffin molds (preferably made of silicone) and bake for 30 - 35 minutes at 200 degrees, until the dough no longer trickles in the mold and has a firm shape.

Nutritional information / 1 serving

- Calories 48 Kcal
- carbohydrates 1 g
- Fiber   0 g
- Proteins 8 g
- Fat 2 g

DAIRY FREE BLACK BEAN BROWNIES WITH CRANBERRIES, COCONUT AND NUTS

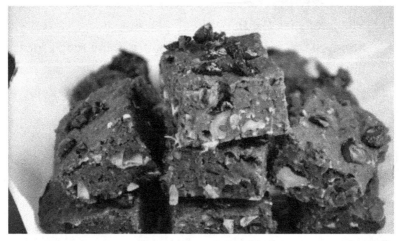

Ingredients for 16 slices

- 300 g cooked black beans (150 g when dry)
- 1 ripe banana
- 1/2 cup cocoa (I recommend this one)
- 1/2 cup of oatmeal (I recommend this one)
- 1/2 cup of dates
- 50 g applesauce
- 2 eggs
- 2 - 4 tbsp honey
- 1 teaspoon vanilla extract
- 70 g dry cranberries (or raisins)
- 50 g desiccated coconut
- 50 g walnuts / pecans (I recommend these)

Preparation time: 40 mins

preparation

1. Mix beans (cooked), oatmeal, banana, cocoa, dates, eggs, honey, vanilla extract and applesauce in the food processor until smooth.
2. Finally add the dry cranberries, desiccated coconut and nuts (chopped into pieces) to the batter.
3. Put the finished dough in the baking pan lined with baking paper and bake for 35 minutes at 180 degrees.
4. The brownies can be served warm, but they still taste delicious after being stored in the refrigerator.

Nutritional information / 1 slice

- Calories 126 Kcal
- carbohydrates 16 g
- Fiber 4 g
- Proteins 5 g
- Fat 4 g

BANANA MUFFINS

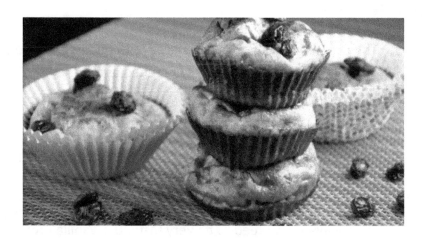

Ingredients for 5 servings

- 1 large banana
- 2 eggs
- 1 scoop (30 g) protein powder

Preparation time: 25 mins

preparation

1. The protein powder can be replaced with pudding powder, dry milk or almond flour and sweetened as required.
2. Mix all ingredients in a blender. Divide the batter into the muffin tins (fill about half of the tin) and bake for 15-20 minutes at 190 degrees until browned.
3. The final consistency of the muffins also depends on the protein powder used.
4. Sometimes they can be firmer, other times softer, but they are always guaranteed to be very tasty. Use vanilla protein concentrate for best results.

Nutritional information / 1 serving

- Calories 67 Kcal
- carbohydrates 5 g
- Fiber   1 g
- Proteins 6 g
- Fat 2 g

SPINACH CAKES WITH CHICKEN

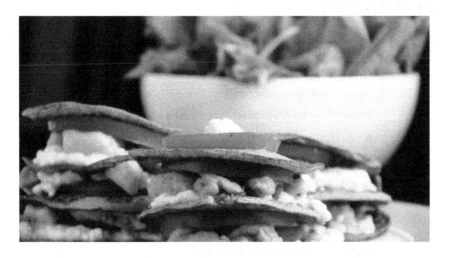

Ingredients for 2 servings

For the cakes:

- 100 g fresh spinach
- 40 g oatmeal (I recommend this one)
- 3 large egg whites
- 40 g yogurt

For the filling:

- 250 g of chicken
- 100 g cottage cheese or fresh mozzarella (sliced)
- 1 tomato
- basil

Preparation time: 30 mins

preparation

1. Cut the chicken breast into pieces and grill in a pan. Then cover them so they don't get cold.
2. Puree all the ingredients for the spinach cakes in a blender as smoothly as possible. Then put the dough in the heated pan so that small cakes are formed and fry each cake for about 1 minute on each side.
3. Either stack the finished cakes in towers or serve them according to your imagination.
4. The chicken in this recipe can of course be replaced with other meat or omitted entirely.

Nutritional information / 1 serving

- Calories 307 Kcal
- carbohydrates 13 g
- Fiber 3 g
- Proteins 49 g
- Fat 5 g

DAIRY-FREE CHOCOLATE SHAKE

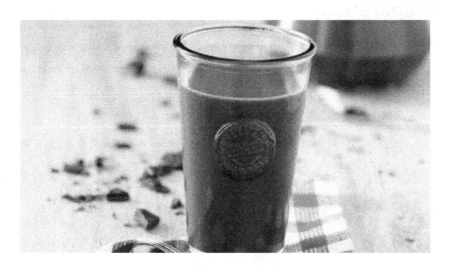

Ingredients for 4 servings

- 1 small banana
- 1 ripe avocado
- 700 ml rice or almond drink
- 1 teaspoon coconut oil
- 3 tbsp cocoa
- Vanilla to taste
- Rice syrup or agave syrup if necessary

Preparation time: 10 mins

preparation

1. Halve the avocado, remove the core and skin, cut into small pieces and put in a blender together with the peeled, chopped up banana and rice drink (or almond drink) and process to a creamy mass.
2. Then add the remaining ingredients and mix well again, season to taste, if necessary (if the shake is too thick) add a little rice drink.
3. Fill into glasses and serve.

Nutritional information / 1 serving

- Calories 407 Kcal
- carbohydrates 24 g
- Fiber 3 g
- Proteins 32 g
- Fat 8 g

SHARON FRUIT AND BANANA SMOOTHIE SHAKES

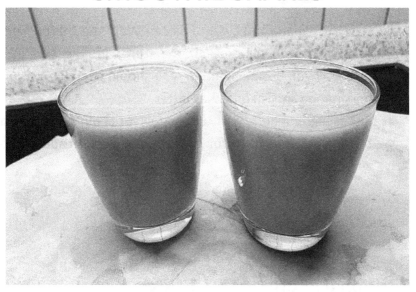

Ingredients for 2 servings

- 1 Sharon fruit or persimmon, ripe
- 1 small Banana (s), ripe
- 1 tsp, leveled   Forest honey
- 160 g Coconut yogurt (yogurt alternative)
- 120 ml orange juice
- 100 ml Oat drink or almond drink
- 0.33 tsp cinnamon
- ¼ tsp turmeric

Preparation time: 10 mins

preparation

1. Peel the banana and cut into pieces. Wash the Sharon fruit, remove the flower and cut the fruit with the skin into pieces. If you use persimmon, you should peel the fruit, as persimmon shells are rather bitter.
2. Put all ingredients in a mixer and mix for about 1 minute on the highest level. If it is too thick for you, you can add a little vegetable milk.
3. The recipe makes 2 small glasses. Vegans should use an appropriate sweetener instead of honey.

Nutritional information / 1 serving

- Calories 215 Kcal
- carbohydrates 16 g
- Fiber 7 g
- Proteins 28 g
- Fat 3 g

Easy risotto with beetroot and goat cheese

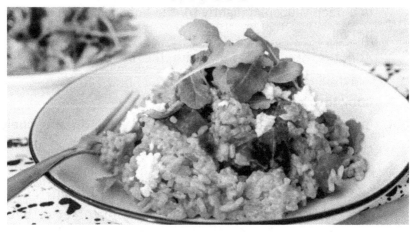

Ingredients for 4 servings

- 2 cups of rice
- 4 cups of vegetable stock
- 250g cooked beetroot
- 2 onions
- 1 tbsp olive oil
- 200g soft goat cheese
- sea-salt
- ground black pepper

Preparation

Preparation 30 minutes

1. In a deep saucepan, lightly fry the finely chopped onion in hot oil.
2. Add the rice, fry briefly with the onion and pour the vegetable stock on top.
3. Cook the rice until soft.
4. Before the rice has finished cooking, mix in the finely chopped, cooked beetroot.
5. As soon as the rice is ready, mix in the goat cheese.
6. Season the risotto with salt and ground black pepper.
7. The risotto can be served sprinkled with rocket or baby spinach. You can also serve it with braised salmon, for example.

Nutritional information / 1 serving

- Calories   298 Kcal
- carbohydrates 29 g
- Fiber   4 g
- Proteins   13 g
- fat   15 g

Healthy raspberry cheesecake in a glass

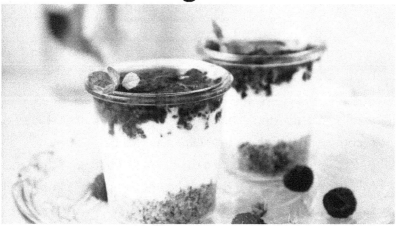

Ingredients for 4 servings

- 100g pecans / walnuts (I recommend these)
- 1 tbsp honey
- 1/2 teaspoon cinnamon
- 600g low-fat Greek yogurt (or quark)
- 4 tbsp honey or xylitol
- 1 teaspoon vanilla extract
- 2 cups (250g) raspberries

Preparation

Preparation 15 minutes

1. Mix the nuts, a tablespoon of honey and cinnamon in a food processor.
2. Divide the resulting, crumbly dough and press it on the bottom of 4 glasses or bowls.
3. Mix the yogurt (or quark) with 4 tablespoons of honey and vanilla extract in a bowl. For an even better taste, I recommend whipping the filling for a while.
4. Pour the filling evenly onto the prepared batter in the jars.
5. Mix the raspberries with 2 tablespoons of water in a small saucepan and cook them until soft.
6. Let the raspberries cool for a while, then pour them over the cheesecakes.
7. The cheesecake can be served straight away or you can let it sit in the refrigerator for a few hours.

Nutritional information / 1 serving

- Calories   352 Kcal
- carbohydrates 35 g
- Fiber   7 g
- Proteins   18 g
- fat   15 g

Simple pasta with beetroot pesto

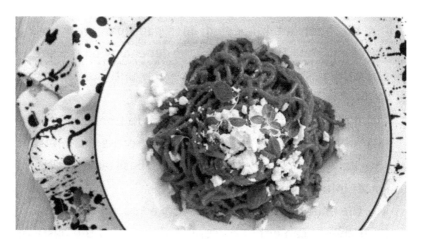

Ingredients for 4 servings

- 500g whole wheat pasta (e.g., spaghetti)
- 2 medium-sized beets
- 1 small handful of fresh basil leaves
- 1-2 tbsp olive oil
- 100g goat (or sheep) cheese
- 50g walnuts (or pine nuts) (I recommend these)
- Juice of 1/2 lemon
- 2 cloves of garlic
- Salt, ground black pepper (to taste)

Preparation

Preparation 70 minutes

1. Put the beetroot (unpeeled) in a saucepan with boiling water and cook for 40-60 minutes depending on the size.
2. Cook the pasta in boiling, salted water until soft and then drain.
3. Clean the cooked beetroot and cut it into smaller pieces.
4. In a food processor or other blender, process the beetroot with garlic, lemon juice, nuts, olive oil, basil leaves, salt and spices into a smooth dough.
5. Mix the finished pesto with the cooked pasta.
6. Goat cheese can either be sprinkled on top of the pasta or mixed under the pasta so that it melts and the pasta becomes even creamier.

Nutritional information / 1 serving

- Calories   678 Kcal
- carbohydrates 86 g
- Fiber   12 g
- Proteins   26 g
- fat   21 g

Simple Greek salad

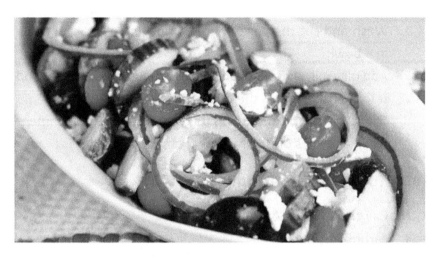

Ingredients for 2 servings

- 200g cherry tomatoes
- 1 cucumber
- 70g feta cheese
- 70g Kalamata olives
- 1/2 red onion
- 1-2 tbsp extra virgin olive oil
- 1 teaspoon of wine vinegar
- ground black pepper

Preparation

Preparation 10 minutes

1. Wash and cut the vegetables, onions and olives and place in a bowl.
2. Add olive oil, wine vinegar, freshly ground black pepper and feta cheese and mix the ingredients well.
3. The salad can be served on its own, as an accompaniment to meat dishes or to wholemeal bread.

Nutritional information / 1 serving

- Calories   180 Kcal
- carbohydrates 8 g
- Fiber   3 g
- Proteins   7 g
- fat   13 g

Spelled chocolate crêpes with ricotta and hot raspberries

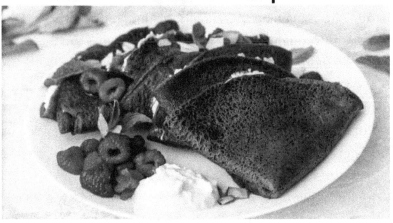

Ingredients for 4 servings

For the crêpes:

- 600ml milk
- 250g fine wholemeal spelled flour (or whole wheat flour)
- 3 tbsp cocoa powder (I recommend this one)
- 2 eggs
- a pinch of salt
- For the filling:
- 150g ricotta (low fat)
- 200g quark (or low-fat cream cheese)
- 2 tbsp honey / maple syrup
- 2 tbsp desiccated coconut
- 1 teaspoon vanilla extract (or vanilla pod)
- 250g frozen raspberries

Preparation

Preparation 30 minutes

1. Mix the spelled flour with cocoa and a pinch of salt in a bowl.
2. Add the remaining ingredients of the crepes and mix the batter thoroughly with a whisk. If the dough is too thin, add a little more flour (the consistency may vary depending on the flour used) and vice versa, if it is too thick, add a little more milk or water.
3. Put the finished dough in portions in a heated non-stick pan (if necessary, oil lightly at the beginning) and fry the crepes on both sides until golden yellow.
4. In the meantime, mix all the ingredients for the filling (except for the raspberries) in a bowl.
5. Spread the resulting cream on the prepared crêpes and then fold / roll them up and place on a plate.
6. Heat the raspberries and pour them over the prepared pancakes.

Nutritional information / 1 serving

- Calories   490 Kcal
- carbohydrates 60 g
- Fiber   14 g
- Proteins   28 g
- fat   10 g

Baked millet with mushrooms and sardines

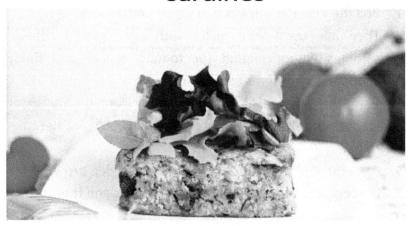

Ingredients for 2 servings

- 1/2 cup of millet
- 3/4 cup of water
- 300g mushrooms
- 2 eggs
- 150g sardines (e.g. in water or oil)
- 40 g grated mozzarella
- 1/2 onion

Preparation

Preparation 55 minutes

1. Boil the millet in a 3/4 cup of water until tender.
2. Then mix the boiled millet with eggs, grated cheese, sardines without liquid (or tomato sauce) and finely chopped mushrooms and onions.
3. Pour the mixture into a parchment-lined baking sheet (choose the size depending on how tall you want the cake to be).
4. Bake for 40-45 minutes at 180 ° C until golden brown.
5. Let cool for at least 5 minutes after baking and then cut.

Nutritional information / 1 serving

- Calories   355 Kcal
- carbohydrates 14 g
- Fiber   3 g
- Proteins   35 g
- fat   17 g

Sweet potato ice cream with chocolate oat balls

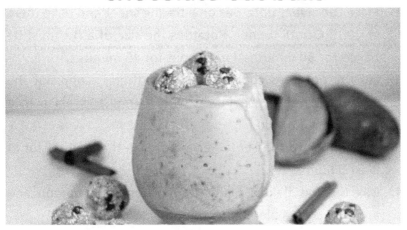

Ingredients for 2 servings

- 250 g sweet potatoes (2 smaller ones)
- 1 cup of milk (any)
- 30g dates
- a pinch of cinnamon
- a spoonful of protein powder (optional) (I recommend this one)

for the balls:

- 70g oatmeal (I recommend this one)
- 40g cashew nuts (I recommend this one)
- 2 tbsp honey
- 2 tbsp applesauce
- 20g dark chocolate chips (I recommend these)
- a pinch of cinnamon
-

Preparation

Preparation 45 minutes

1. Place the sweet potatoes on a baking sheet and bake them at 200 ° C until tender. Potatoes the size of a fist must be baked for 30 minutes, larger ones for 45 minutes.
2. Let the potatoes cool and then cut them, scoop out the inside and mash the inside with a fork and place in a container with a lid.
3. Pour milk into the container and freeze the mixture for at least 5 hours.
4. Mix the oat flakes, cashew nuts, honey, cinnamon and applesauce in a blender as smoothly as possible.
5. Add the chocolate chips to the oat mixture and shape into small balls. Keep in the refrigerator until the ice cream is served.
6. Before serving, take the frozen mixture out of the freezer, let it thaw for 5 minutes, and mix it with the other ingredients to form a smooth ice cream. If this is very difficult, put some fresh milk in the blender.
7. If you don't like the taste of sweet potatoes, I recommend adding a spoonful of protein powder.
8. Serve the ice cream in bowls, garnish with the balls and serve immediately.

Nutritional information / 1 serving

- Calories   195 Kcal
- carbohydrates 38 g
- Fiber   4 g
- Proteins   5 g

Roasted "Caprese" chicken breast with tomatoes, basil and mozzarella

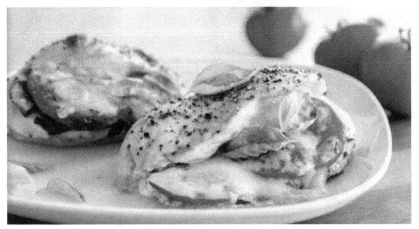

Ingredients for 4 servings

- 800g (4 medium-sized pieces) chicken breast
- 200g fresh mozzarella
- a handful of fresh basil
- 2 tomatoes
- ground black pepper (to taste)
- Salt (to taste)
- Garlic powder (to taste)
- Balsamic vinegar (optional)
- 1-2 tbsp olive oil

Preparation

Preparation 35 minutes

1. Cut the chicken breast on one side. The other side should be kept closed to prevent the ingredients from falling out.
2. Drizzle the meat on both sides with olive oil and massage in the spices and salt by hand depending on your taste.
3. Cut tomatoes and mozzarella into thin slices.
4. Place a few slices of mozzarella and tomatoes in each piece of meat. Also add basil leaves.
5. Place the stuffed chicken breasts in a baking dish.
6. Bake the meat (can be covered) in the preheated oven at 220 degrees Celsius for about 20 minutes until it is cooked through. After baking, let it sit in a covered pan for at least 5 minutes.
7. Finally, you can add balsamic vinegar and serve it with your favorite side dish.

Nutritional information / 1 serving

-   Calories   403 Kcal
-   carbohydrates 3 g
-   Fiber   1 g
-   Proteins   55 g
-   fat   16 g

Low carbohydrate tomato frittata

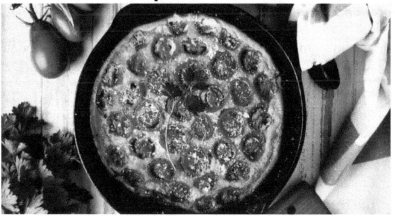

Ingredients for 2 servings

- 4 large eggs
- 2 Table spoons of milk
- 2 tbsp tomato puree
- 3 tbsp grated parmesan cheese
- 250g cherry tomatoes
- 1 teaspoon olive oil
- ground black pepper
- 1/2 teaspoon sea salt

Preparation

Preparation 15 minutes

1. In a bowl, mix the eggs, milk, tomato puree, sea salt, ground black pepper, and a spoonful of grated Parmesan cheese.
2. Heat the olive oil in a deep pan.
3. Pour the egg mixture into the pan.
4. Cover the pan and simmer over medium heat for 5 minutes, until most of the frittata thickens.
5. Cover the frittata with the chopped cherry tomatoes and the rest of the Parmesan cheese and let cook, covered, for another 5-7 minutes, checking occasionally that it does not burn.

Nutritional information / 1 serving

- Calories   230 Kcal
- carbohydrates 6 g
- Fiber   2 g
- Proteins   17 g
- fat   15 g

Simple baked oat donuts

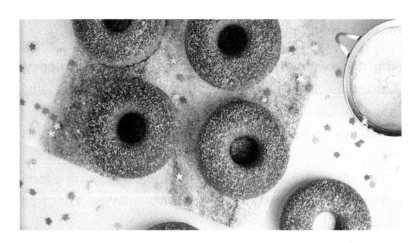

Ingredients for 6 servings

- 1 1/2 cups of finely ground oats (almost made into flour) (I recommend this)
- 12 dates (or 3 tbsp honey)
- 1/2 cup of milk of your choice (125 ml)
- 1 tbsp starch
- 1 teaspoon Baking powder
- 1 teaspoon vanilla extract
- 1 teaspoon cinnamon

Preparation

Preparation 25 minutes

1. Tip: If you want to use dates in your recipe instead of honey, let them soak in warm water for at least 30 minutes and then work them into a smooth paste.
2. First mix the dry ingredients together, then mix in the remaining ingredients.
3. Place the batter in a silicone donut mold. If you use a form other than silicone, lubricate it with a little coconut oil beforehand.
4. Bake the donuts at 180 degrees for 15-18 minutes.
5. For the sugar effect, you can sprinkle the finished donuts with coconut flour or use a frosting of your choice.
6. Donuts can also be served with homemade jam.

Nutritional information / 1 piece

- Calories   114 Kcal
- carbohydrates 21 g
- Fiber   2 g
- Proteins   3 g
- fat   2 g

Low carbohydrate salad wrap

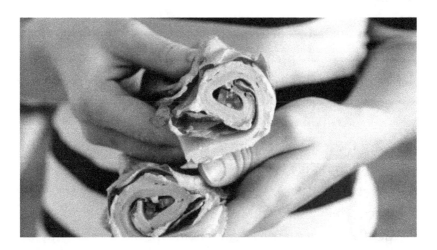

Ingredients for 1 serving

- 2 large lettuce leaves
- 50g high quality ham
- 30g semi-hard cheese (e.g., Swiss cheese)
- 1/4 avocado
- 1/2 tomato
- Pinch of ground black pepper

Preparation

Preparation 5 minutes

1. Wash the lettuce leaves under running water and let them dry.
2. Clean the avocado and mash it with a fork.
3. Mix the avocado puree with a pinch of ground black pepper and spread on one of the lettuce leaves.
4. Place the lettuce leaf with the avocado on a second washed leaf so that they stick together.
5. Cover the lettuce leaves with slices of ham and cheese and place a thinly sliced tomato on top.
6. Gently roll the lettuce leaves with the filling as tightly as possible. You can cut the wrap in half or use a toothpick to hold it in place to keep it from opening.

Nutritional information / 1 serving

- Calories   266 Kcal
- carbohydrates 5 g
- Fiber   4 g
- Proteins   20 g
- fat   18 g

Braised cod in lemon and garlic sauce with celery fries

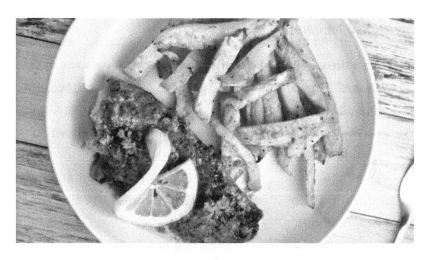

Ingredients for 3 servings

For the fish:

- 600g cod
- 2 tbsp butter
- 1 lemon (juice + zest)
- 2 cloves of garlic
- 1 tbsp mustard
- 1-2 tbsp soy sauce
- parsley

For the celery fries:

- 1kg celery
- 1 teaspoon sea salt
- 1/2 teaspoon paprika
- 1/2 teaspoon marjoram
- 1 tbsp olive oil

Preparation

Preparation 65 minutes

1. Wash the celery and cut into thin fries.
2. Prepare a marinade for french fries in a large bowl. Mix olive oil, spices and salt.
3. Put the sliced french fries in the bowl and cover with the marinade.
4. Place the fries on a parchment-lined baking sheet and bake them for 40 to 50 minutes at 220 degrees, turning them after 20 minutes.
5. In the meantime, prepare the cod in a frying pan. Heat the butter and add the pressed garlic cloves, mustard, lemon juice and zest, soy sauce. Then put the cod in the pan.
6. Cover the pan and simmer the fish over low heat for about 10-15 minutes. Add a little water if necessary.
7. Finally sprinkle the fish with fresh parsley.
8. Serve the fish with baked celery fries, the prepared sauce and, for example, fresh salad.

Nutritional information / 1 serving

- Calories   368 Kcal
- carbohydrates 7 g
- Fiber   6 g
- Proteins   50 g
- fat   12 g

Healthy coconut and apple porridge

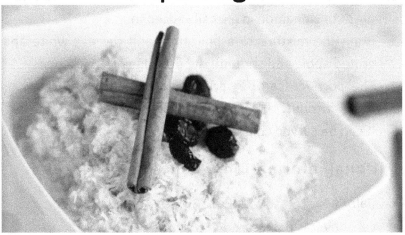

Ingredients for 1 serving

- 1 apple
- 40g (6 tbsp) desiccated coconut
- 1 egg white
- 2 tbsp applesauce
- 1/2 cup coconut milk (or another type of milk)
- a pinch of cinnamon
- Protein powder (optional) (I recommend this one)

Preparation

Preparation 15 minutes

1. Finely grate the apple.
2. Mix the desiccated coconut with milk, apple sauce and a pinch of cinnamon in a small saucepan.
3. Bring the mixture to a boil, then add the egg white and grated apple and stir until the porridge has thickened.
4. The porridge can be sprinkled with nuts, dried fruits or more coconut.
5. It can be served cold or warm.

Nutritional information / 1 serving

- Calories   360 Kcal
- carbohydrates 36 g
- Fiber   4 g
- Proteins   7 g
- fat   21 g

Healthy coconut rolls without baking

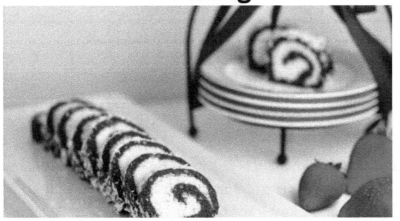

ingredients

- 170g graham crackers (I recommend buckwheat)
- 1-2 tbsp honey
- 2-3 tbsp water
- 1 tbsp cocoa powder (I recommend this one)
- 1 tbsp ground coffee

for the filling:

- 100g coconut
- 1 tbsp honey

Preparation

Preparation 25 minutes

1. Mix the biscuits with flour in a mixer.
2. In a bowl, mix the ground biscuits with honey, cocoa, ground coffee and two tablespoons of water.
3. Knead the dough by hand. If the batter is too hard, add another tablespoon of water.
4. Prepare the coconut filling in a food chopper (small food processor).
5. Mix coconut and honey on high speed for 10-15 minutes with breaks until a buttery mixture (coconut butter) is formed. The longer you blend, the butterier the mixture will be. (I recommend using a food processor and adding some water if the filling doesn't get thicker over time).
6. Roll out the dough between two sheets of parchment paper into a 3 mm square shape and spread the coconut filling evenly over it.
7. Gently roll the dough up (the parchment paper will help) and let it set in the refrigerator for at least 8 hours.
8. Cut the roulade and sprinkle with desiccated coconut.

Nutritional information / 1 slice

- Calories   95 Kcal
- carbohydrates 13 g
- Fiber   1 g
- Proteins   2 g
- fat   4

Pumpkin "spaghetti" with minced turkey in tomato sauce

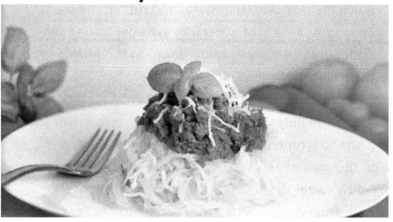

Ingredients for 2 servings

- 1 spaghetti squash
- 300g minced turkey
- 1 onion
- 1 tbsp coconut oil (I recommend this one)
- 200g tomato puree
- 4 cloves of garlic
- 1 teaspoon sea salt
- 1/2 teaspoon of ground black pepper
- basil
- 150ml of water

Preparation

Preparation 60 minutes

1. Halve the pumpkin lengthways and cut out the seeds.
2. Pour approx. 2 cm of water into a deeper baking pan, place both pumpkin halves (inside down) in the form and cover them with perforated aluminum foil.
3. Bake the pumpkin for 45 minutes at 205 ° C.
4. After 45 minutes, remove the pumpkin, turn it over and use a fork to scrape the inside into "spaghetti".
5. In the meantime, melt the coconut oil in a saucepan and lightly sweat the finely chopped onion.
6. Add ground turkey, tomato puree, spices, sea salt and water to the saucepan and stir the mixture thoroughly.
7. Cover and cook the meat for 30 minutes.
8. Add the pressed garlic cloves to the meat, if necessary, a little more water and fresh basil and cook covered for another 5 minutes.
9. Serve the finished meat with pumpkin spaghetti. You can also sprinkle grated cheese on top.

Nutritional information / 1 serving

- Calories   400 kcal
- carbohydrates 25 g
- Fiber   7 g
- Proteins   33 g
- fat   17 g

No-bake fitness chocolate cheesecake

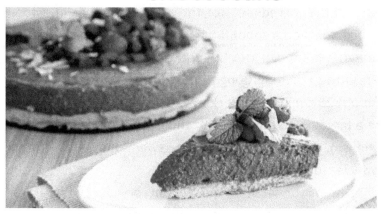

Ingredients for 12 servings

- 600g low-fat natural Greek yogurt (or quark or a mixture of both)
- 400g low-fat cream cheese (such as Philadelphia)
- 100g "Dutch-process" cocoa
- 150g xylitol (or the equivalent of stevia or cane sugar)
- 200g raspberries (for decorating)
- 30g 100% gelatin powder
- 1 scoop of chocolate protein powder (optional) (I recommend this one)
- Mint (to decorate)
- For the dough:
- 200g oatmeal (I recommend this one)
- 2 tbsp honey
- 2 tbsp melted coconut oil (I recommend this one)
- 1-3 tbsp water (as neede

Preparation

Preparation 25 minutes

1. Mix all the ingredients for the dough together in a food processor. Add a spoonful of water as required so that the dough is homogeneous but not too moist.
2. Press the resulting dough onto the bottom of a cake tin (about 25 cm in diameter).
3. In a large bowl, mix together the Greek yogurt (or cottage cheese), cream cheese, cocoa, sweetener, and protein powder (optional).
4. In a small bowl, mix the gelatin powder with a few tablespoons of boiling water. Stir it until it dissolves.
5. Add a few tablespoons of chocolate cream to the melted gelatin and mix them together well.
6. Mix the prepared gelatin mixture with the rest of the chocolate cream.
7. Pour the chocolate cream onto the prepared dough.
8. Put the cheesecake in the refrigerator for at least 5 hours.
9. Decorate the chocolate cheesecake with raspberries and mint.

Nutritional information / 1 slice

- Calories   271 Kcal
- carbohydrates 30 g
- Fiber   6 g
- Proteins   17 g
- fat   11 g

Low-calorie protein roulades

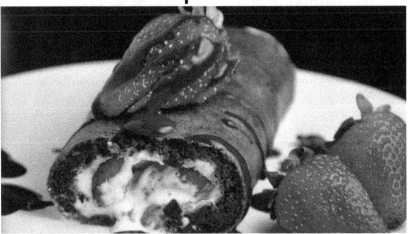

Ingredients for 8 servings

For the dough:

- 4 egg whites
- 2 tbsp cocoa (I recommend this one)
- 1 teaspoon Baking powder
- 1 scoop (30 g) chocolate protein powder (optional) (I recommend this)
- 2 tbsp honey (only if you don't use sweet protein powder)
- 1 pinch of cinnamon

For the filling:

- 120 g quark
- 3 tbsp Greek yogurt
- 50 g strawberries (possibly banana or other fruit)

- 1 scoop (30g) vanilla protein powder (optional) (I recommend this one)
- 2 tbsp honey (only if you don't use sweet protein powder)

Preparation

Preparation 25 minutes

1. Beat the egg whites into snow and then carefully mix in the cocoa, protein powder, cinnamon and baking powder. If you don't use protein powder, add the chosen sweetener.
2. Pour the resulting dough into a square baking pan lined with baking paper and bake for 10-15 minutes at 150 degrees. Let the baked dough cool down.
3. Filling: Mix the quark, yoghurt and protein powder (or the sweetener) in a bowl. Cut the selected fruit into pieces and stir in. If you take bananas, you can put them whole in the roulade. Put the filling on the cooled dough base and roll everything into a roulade. Leave the roulade in the refrigerator for at least 2 hours.

Nutritional information / 1 slice

- Calories   50 Kcal
- carbohydrates 2 g
- Fiber   1 g
- Proteins   9 g
- fat   1 g

REFRESHING, HEALTHY, FROZEN FRUIT PIE

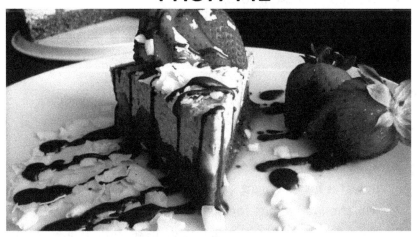

Ingredients for 12 servings

For the colorful layer:

- 2 cups of fruit from the freezer (strawberries / blueberries / blackberries / raspberries)
- 3 ripe bananas
- 1 tbsp coconut oil (I recommend this one)

For the top layer:

- 1 cup of cashew nuts (I recommend this one)
- 1/2 cup almonds (I recommend this one)
- 1 banana
- 1/2 cup dates / raisins / prunes

- 5 tbsp solid coconut milk (solid part on the surface that is created when the coconut milk is left in the refrigerator for one night)
- 5 tbsp soft quark
- 1/2 cup desiccated coconut
- Water as needed (the less, the better)

Preparation

Preparation 20 minutes

1. Soak cashew nuts and almonds (or dates, if you take them) in water for one night.
2. Mix the ingredients for the colored layer in the mixer and then put them in a mold (e.g. cake tin). Place in the refrigerator for 30 to 60 minutes.
3. Now prepare the top part of the cake. Mix all the ingredients for the upper part of the cake in the mixer until smooth. If the mixture is difficult to mix, add a little water - the less, the better.
4. Take the colored part of the cake out of the freezer as soon as it is stiff on top. Now, if necessary, distribute fruit on top and cover with the top layer.
5. Put the prepared cake in the freezer for one night. Take it out of the freezer at least 1 hour before serving to soften it. It can be stored in the refrigerator for a maximum of half a day, then it will start to melt. Before serving, you can decorate them with strawberries, pour melted dark chocolate over them or sprinkle with desiccated coconut. Store in the freezer.

Nutritional information / 1 slice

- Calories   185 Kcal
- carbohydrates 14 g
- Fiber   3 g
- Proteins   5 g
- fat   13 g

CHOCOLATE MUG WITH PEANUT BUTTER

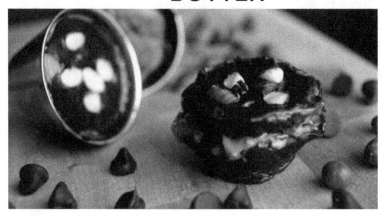

Ingredients for 4 servings

- 3 tbsp coconut oil (I recommend this one)
- 2 tbsp cocoa (I recommend this one)
- 6 tbsp chocolate chips (70% or higher) (I recommend this)
- 4 tbsp peanut butter (I recommend this one)
- grated almonds / coconut for crumble

Preparation

Preparation 10 minutes

1. Melt the coconut oil together with the chocolate chips and cocoa in a small saucepan with a non-stick layer (if you like it sweeter, add 1 tbsp agave syrup or honey or a little stevia). Mix smoothly. Remove from heat and pour into the prepared bowls / baskets / muffin tins (approx. 1 tbsp mixture per basket).
2. Let it cool down briefly and set and pour the peanut butter (1 spoon per cup) on this layer.
3. Pour the rest of the chocolate mixture over it, sprinkle with almonds or desiccated coconut if necessary and put in the refrigerator for one night.
4. If you get an appetite for chocolate, just take it out of the fridge and eat :)

Nutritional information / 1 serving

- Calories   271 Kcal
- carbohydrates 13 g
- Fiber   4 g
- Proteins   5 g
- fat   24 g

Protein curd dumplings

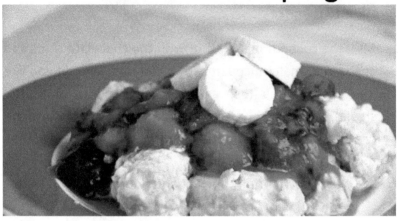

Ingredients for 1 serving

- 250 g crumb quark
- 1 egg
- 20 g protein powder (preferably sweetened with natural flavor and stevia) (I recommend this)
- 3 - 5 tbsp oat flour (or chickpea, whole grain or spelled semolina flour) (I recommend this)
- 150 g strawberries (or other fruit)

Preparation

Preparation 15 minutes

1. Mix the quark, protein powder, flour and egg thoroughly in a bowl.
2. First add only 3 tablespoons of flour to the dough.
3. If it is too thin, add more flour.
4. Shape the finished dough into balls with the help of spoons and add them to boiling water.
5. Wait for the dumplings to float on top and cook for another 2 minutes.
6. Sieve the finished dumplings and serve with mashed strawberries or other fruit.
7. If you don't have protein powder available, don't worry: you can prepare the dumplings without them - you can replace them with two more spoons of flour.

Nutritional information / 1 serving

- Calories   440 kcal
- carbohydrates 27 g
- Fiber   4 g
- Proteins   64 g
- fat   8 g

Lean cabbage gnocchi

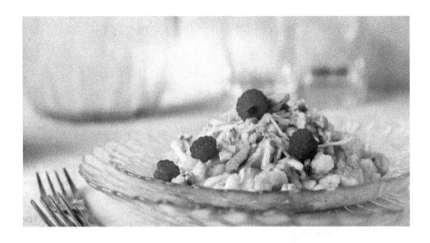

Ingredients for 2 servings

- ½ cabbage
- 1 apple
- 40 g ground nuts (I recommend this one)
- 100 g quark
- 2 tbsp honey
- cinnamon
- Fruit / nuts / desiccated coconut / poppy seeds (optional)
- Raisins / cranberries (optional)

Preparation

Preparation 15 minutes

1. Cut the cabbage into small pieces and cook in the boiling water for about 7-10 minutes.
2. Then mix in a bowl with the grated apple, cinnamon and sweetener and serve sprinkled with nuts, quark and possibly other sprinkles.

Nutritional information / 1 serving

- Calories   298 Kcal
- carbohydrates 28 g
- Fiber   10 g
- Proteins   18 g
- fat   10 g

Simple potato soup with mushrooms & tuna

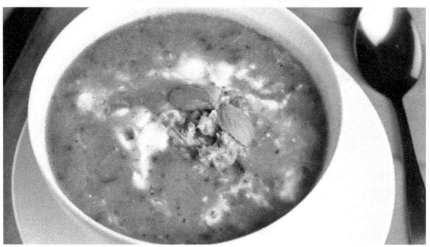

Ingredients for 4 servings

- 500 g mushrooms
- 1 onion
- 2 medium-sized potatoes
- 2 cloves of garlic
- 2 L (8 cups) chicken stock (or water)
- 1 teaspoon salt
- 1 pinch of black pepper (ground)
- 1 tbsp butter
- 150 g tuna in its own juice (optional)
- 4 tbsp Greek yogurt (to thicken after cooking - optional)

Preparation

Preparation 30 minutes

1. Peel the onion and chop finely.
2. Wash and finely chop the mushrooms.
3. Heat a spoonful of butter in a non-stick saucepan and lightly fry the chopped onions.
4. Add the mushrooms and sauté, stirring occasionally, until tender (about 5 minutes).
5. Add the chicken broth or water and bring the soup to a boil.
6. In the meantime, mix the finely chopped raw potatoes with 2 cloves of garlic and a little water with a mixer.
7. Add the mixture to the soup.
8. Let the soup boil for about 10-15 minutes and then puree with a hand blender and then season with salt and pepper.
9. If desired, stir in the Greek yogurt before serving. I also recommend adding some drained tuna. This gives the soup a protein kick and it also tastes really delicious.

Nutritional information / 1 serving

- Calories   135 Kcal
- carbohydrates 18 g
- Fiber   5 g
- Proteins   7 g
- fat   4 g

Healthy homemade crunchy muesli made from oats, buckwheat and quinoa

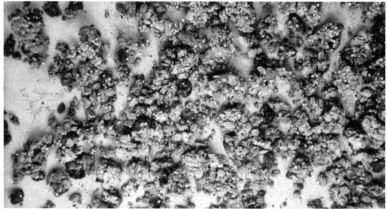

Ingredients for 5 servings

- 1 cup of oatmeal (I recommend this one)
- 1/2 cup dried buckwheat
- 1/4 cup dried quinoa
- 3 tbsp chia seeds (I recommend these)
- 5 tbsp protein powder (or dry milk powder) (I recommend this one)
- 3-4 tbsp melted coconut oil (I recommend this one)
- 3 tbsp applesauce
- 1-2 tablespoons of honey
- 1 teaspoon vanilla extract
- Raisins, cranberries, nuts, coconut, dark chocolate pieces (as you like) (I recommend these)

Preparation

Preparation 50 minutes

1. Mix all ingredients in a bowl.
2. Then spread in a thin layer on a baking sheet lined with baking paper.
3. Bake the muesli for 35-45 minutes at 165 degrees Celsius, checking and turning every 10 minutes.
4. If the oven has a high heat output and the muesli is too dark, simply take it out of the oven after 30-35 minutes.
5. Allow the baked granola to cool completely on the baking tray (it will harden), then break it into pieces and place in a sealed container for storage.

Nutritional information / 1 serving

- Calories   280 Kcal
- carbohydrates 30 g
- Fiber   6 g
- Proteins   11 g
- fat   12 g

Flaxseed Pizza Dough

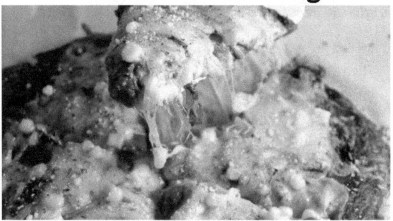

Ingredients for 2 servings

- 1 cup of ground flaxseed (I recommend this one)
- 2 eggs
- 50 g of grated cheese
- Topping (to taste)

Preparation

Preparation 30 minutes

1. Grind the flax seeds (use ground ones from the shop if necessary) and mix with the eggs and cheese.
2. Line the baking sheet with parchment paper and spread the dough on it in a circle.
3. This circle should measure approx. 25 cm in diameter so that the pizza base does not get too thin.
4. Bake the dough in the oven at 175 degrees.
5. Take out after about 8 minutes and top with the desired ingredients.
6. Bake for another 15 minutes.

Nutritional information / 1 serving

- Calories   542 Kcal
- carbohydrates 6 g
- Fiber   22 g
- Proteins   30 g
- fat   36 g

Raspberry cake with avocado cocoa filling

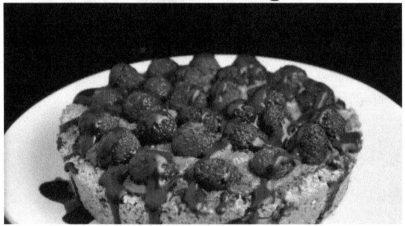

Ingredients for 8 servings

- 1.5 cups of oatmeal (I recommend this one)
- 30 g pecans
- 2 tbsp desiccated coconut
- 3 tbsp honey
- ¼ cup applesauce
- 1 tbsp coconut oil (I recommend this one)
- 1 teaspoon cinnamon
- 150 g raspberries

For the filling:

- 1 ripe avocado
- 250 g Greek yogurt
- 40 g hazelnuts
- ¼ cup of cocoa (I recommend this one)
- 5 tbsp honey

Preparation

Preparation 30 minutes

1. Mix the oat flakes with the nuts almost into flour.
2. Then add desiccated coconut, cinnamon, melted coconut oil, honey and applesauce and mix everything together.
3. Spread the resulting dough on the base and on the edge of a smaller cake tin.
4. Bake the cake base for 10-15 minutes at 190 degrees until golden brown.
5. Filling: Fry the hazelnuts in a dry pan until golden brown and then mix together with the other ingredients until smooth.
6. Spread the filling on the cooled cake base, decorate with raspberries and put in the fridge for at least 3 hours.
7. Finally, you can pour melted dark chocolate over the cake and decorate it with peppermint.

Nutritional information / 1 slice

- Calories   270 Kcal
- carbohydrates 32 g
- Fiber   6 g
- Proteins   8 g
- fat   13 g

Almond cupcakes with coffee and cashew cream

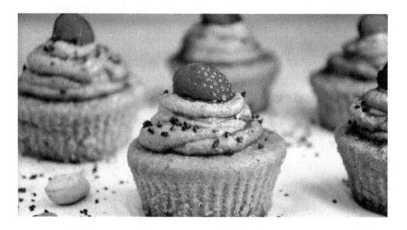

Ingredients for 6 servings

- 4 tbsp ground almonds (I recommend this one)
- 1 egg
- 2 tbsp almond / peanut butter (I recommend this)
- 3 tbsp honey
- ½ cup of milk
- ½ teaspoon baking powder
- 1 pinch of cinnamon
- ¼ cup of cocoa (optional) (I recommend this one)

For the cream:

- 50 g cashew nuts (I recommend this one)
- ½ teaspoon of coffee
- 2 tbsp Greek yogurt
- 2 - 3 tbsp honey
- 1 tbsp cocoa (I recommend this)

Preparation

Preparation 35 minutes

1. In a bowl, mix the ground (or flour) almonds with baking powder, cinnamon and cocoa (for cocoa cupcakes).
2. Then add the other ingredients for the cupcakes to the bowl and mix the dough until it is smooth.
3. Spread the finished dough in silicone muffin molds.
4. This amount should make about 6 large or 12 small cupcakes.
5. Bake for 17-25 minutes at 175 degrees until golden brown.
6. Let cool down well and only then take it out of the mold.
7. Soak the cashew nuts in water for 30-60 minutes.
8. Then rinse and mix in a blender with the other ingredients for the cream.
9. Pour the cream into the cream syringe and decorate the cupcakes.
10. Then top with raspberries and sprinkle with coffee (optional).

Nutritional information / 1 serving

- Calories   175 Kcal
- carbohydrates 19 g
- Fiber   2 g
- Proteins   6 g
- fat   10 g

No-bake banana quark dessert

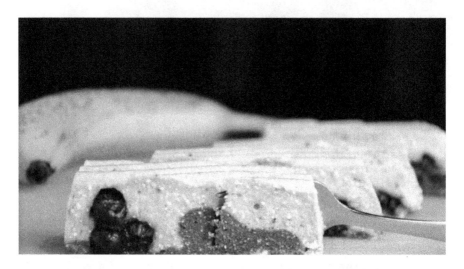

Ingredients for 8 servings

- 2 bananas
- 300 g fine quark
- 2 tbsp gelatin powder
- 100 ml of hot water
- 1 tbsp cocoa (I recommend this)
- 1 tbsp honey
- 100 g soft fruit (can also be from the freezer)

Preparation

Preparation 10 minutes

1. Mix the bananas and quark in a blender.
2. Add the gelatine powder, dissolved in 100 ml hot water, and mix again.
3. When the batter is smooth, pour half of it into a container / mold and let it set for a moment.
4. The taller the dessert should be, the smaller the shape should be.
5. Put a spoonful of cocoa and a spoonful of honey (or other sweetener) in the other half of the batter and mix well again.
6. Pour the finished cocoa dough on the first layer, sprinkle with fresh fruit and place in the refrigerator for at least 5 hours.

Nutritional information / 1 slice

- Calories   80 Kcal
- carbohydrates 10 g
- Fiber   2 g
- Proteins   9 g
- fat   0 g

Homemade chickpea flour

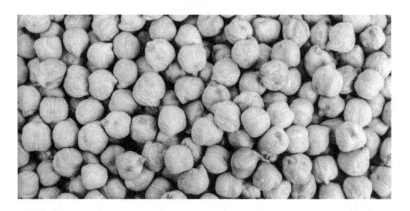

Ingredients for 1 serving

- 100g chickpeas

Preparation

Preparation 10 minutes

1. The chickpea is one of the tastiest legumes and has a subtle nut taste. Chickpeas are high in protein and fiber, and a perfect source of B vitamins, iron, potassium, and magnesium. Chickpeas are not only suitable for healthy people and athletes, but are particularly recommended for these diseases: high cholesterol levels, arteriosclerosis, diabetes, constipation, disorders of the immune system and cancer. Chickpeas do not contain gluten and are therefore also suitable for people with celiac disease. They should be an integral part of any diet. Chickpeas are particularly suitable for children and pregnant women because, unlike other legumes, you hardly feel bloated.

2. Other positive aspects are the nutritional value and the concentration of amino acids in chickpeas - these substances work against cancer. They have a positive effect

on the fats in the body, lower the cholesterol level in the blood and have a beneficial effect on the skin. Thanks to their mineral content, they also help to eliminate mental fatigue, lower blood pressure and have a positive effect on heart activity.

3. By adding chickpea flour when cooking or baking, you increase the biological value of the dish. In many recipes you can replace part of the normal flour with chickpea flour, but in this book you will find many recipes that only recommend chickpea flour.

4. To make homemade chickpea flour, you need a high-quality mixer, food chopper or grinder (e.g. also a coffee grinder).

5. Mix the dry chickpeas in small amounts into flour. Sieve the ground chickpeas at least twice so that all larger parts are found and sorted out. The smoother the flour, the finer the dough will be.

6. Store the flour in an airtight container in the refrigerator.

7. A cup of dry chickpeas is a little less than a cup of chickpea flour.

Note: If you are not lucky with the flour production, you can buy high-quality chickpea flour on the Internet or in health food stores

Nutritional information / 1 serving

- Calories   387 Kcal
- carbohydrates 57 g

- Fiber   10 g
- Proteins   23 g
- fat   7 g

Tuna Couscous Salad

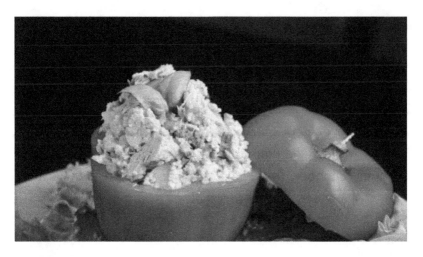

Ingredients for 1 serving

- 150 g tuna in its own juice
- 1/4 cup couscous
- 1/4 onion
- fresh basil
- Sea salt, pepper (to taste)

Preparation

Preparation 10 minutes

1. Cut the onion into small pieces and place in a saucepan with the couscous.
2. Add ½ cup of water, season with salt and pepper and cook until the couscous has completely absorbed the water.
3. Mix the cooked couscous with the (juiced) tuna and the finely chopped fresh basil and serve warm with lettuce, paprika or other fresh vegetables.

Nutritional information / 1 serving

- Calories   275 Kcal
- carbohydrates 28 g
- Fiber   2 g
- Proteins   34 g
- fat   2 g

Fruit curd casserole

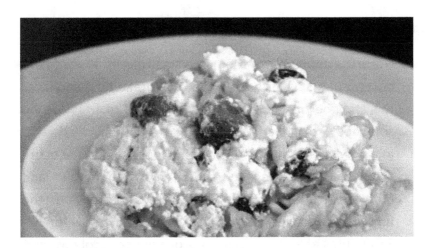

Ingredients for 2 servings

- 2 smaller apples
- 200 g strawberries (or other fruit)
- 2 bananas
- 200 g quark
- 150 g yogurt
- Nuts, raisins, desiccated coconut etc. (optional)
- Cinnamon (optional)
- 1 egg (optional)

Preparation

Preparation 40 minutes

1. Grate the apples or cut them into small pieces. Place on the bottom of a smaller baking pan (e.g. bread box) and layer the strawberries or other fruit on top. The fruit can be sprinkled with cinnamon.

2. In a bowl, mash the bananas with a fork and add the quark and yogurt. Mix the mass thoroughly. You can also add nuts, desiccated coconut or raisins - to taste. Pour the finished quark over the fruit and bake the casserole for 30 - 35 minutes at 180 degrees. Take out the casserole when it turns brown on top and serve either warm or cold.

3. The finished casserole won't hold its shape, but it's delicious! If you want it to keep its shape, add an egg to the quark topping.

Nutritional information / 1 serving

- Calories   367 Kcal
- carbohydrates 57 g
- Fiber   10 g
- Proteins   28 g
- fat   1 g

Carrot and parsley spaghetti with basil pesto

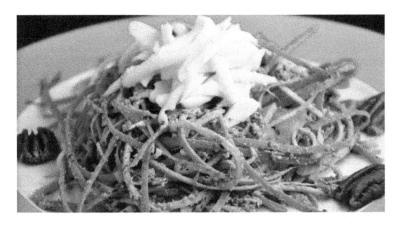

Ingredients for 4 servings

- 500 g carrots
- 250 g parsley
- 100 g cheese (optional)
- For the pesto:
- 2 cloves of garlic
- 1/4 cup walnuts (I recommend this one)
- 2 cups of fresh basil
- 1/2 cup of olive oil
- 1/2 cup of grated parmesan
- Sea salt and pepper (to taste)

Preparation

Preparation 15 minutes

1. Grate the carrots and parsley into spaghetti with a grater or a peeler.
2. Mix all ingredients for the pesto except pepper and salt together in the mixer as smoothly as possible.
3. Finally, season with sea salt and pepper.
4. Mix the finished pesto with the prepared vegetables, possibly sprinkle with grated cheese and serve.
5. Store the remaining pesto in the refrigerator in a sealed container.

Nutritional information / 1 serving

- Calories   445 Kcal
- carbohydrates 10 g
- Fiber   6 g
- Proteins   10 g
- fat   40 g

BAKED WATERMELON WITH MOZZARELLA AND NUTS

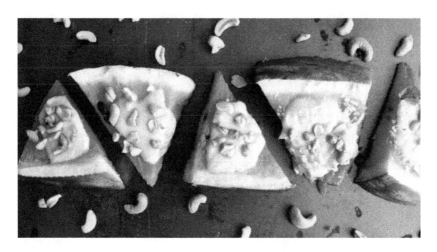

Ingredients for 10 servings

- 400 g watermelon
- 40 g mozzarella
- 40 g nuts (pine nuts / cashew nuts / pistachios / desiccated coconut) (I recommend these)

Preparation

Preparation 15 minutes

1. Preheat the oven to 170 degrees.
2. Cut the melon into triangles and place on a baking pan.
3. Place a piece of mozzarella on each triangle and sprinkle with chopped nuts.
4. Bake for 8-10 minutes, until the mozzarella is at least partially melted.
5. Take out of the oven, season with pepper if necessary and let cool down briefly.

Nutritional information / 1 slice

- Calories   45 Kcal
- carbohydrates 4 g
- Fiber   1 g
- Proteins   2 g
- fat   3 g

COCONUT CUTS WITH EGG YOLK PUDDING

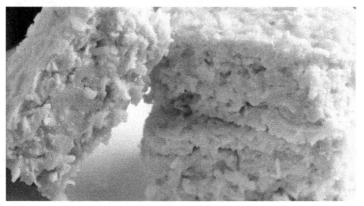

Ingredients for 8 servings

For the dough:

- 5 egg whites
- 1.5 cups desiccated coconut
- 3 tbsp honey

For the filling:

- 5 egg yolks
- 1/2 pack of gelatin powder
- 5 tbsp water
- 1.5 cups of milk
- 3 tbsp honey
- 1 tbsp vanilla flavor
- 3 tbsp chickpea flour
- 3 tbsp yogurt
- 3 tbsp desiccated coconut

Preparation

Preparation 25 minutes

1. First prepare the dough. Mix the egg whites in a bowl with the desiccated coconut and honey (or another sweetener). With this recipe there is no need to beat the egg whites. Pour the resulting dough into the baking pan lined with baking paper. Bake for 20 minutes at 175 degrees until golden brown.
2. Prepare the egg yolk pudding while it is baking. Mix the gelatin powder with 5 tablespoons of water and allow to swell. Then add egg yolks, honey (or other sweetener) and vanilla flavoring and stir thoroughly. Add the milk, mixed with the chickpea flour, and cook the resulting mixture, stirring constantly. When the pudding starts to boil, add desiccated coconut. After 3 minutes, remove the pudding from the stove and stir in the yogurt. This refines the pudding taste.
3. Now cut the dough, which has cooled down after baking, in half and place one half in a smaller container / dish. Spread the egg yolk pudding on this layer and cover with the other half of the batter. Place in a sealed container in the refrigerator for a night or at least 7 hours and allow to set.

Nutritional information / 1 slice

- Calories   170 kcal
- carbohydrates 17 g
- Fiber   2 g
- Proteins   7 g

Tuna salad with cottage cheese, corn and walnuts

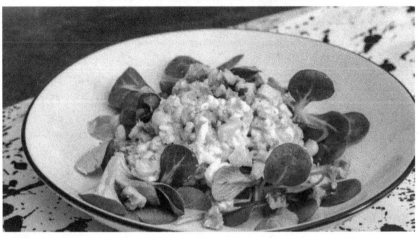

Ingredients for 1 serving

- 150 g tuna in its own juice
- 30 g corn
- 100 g of cottage cheese
- 20 g walnuts (I recommend this one)
- salad
- 1 pinch of paprika powder
- 1 pinch of ground pepper
- 1 pinch of garlic spice
- 1 pinch of sea salt

Preparation

Preparation 5 minutes

1. Cut the lettuce into small pieces and place on a plate.
2. Mix the tuna (juiced) with the cottage cheese, corn and spices in a bowl.
3. Add walnuts and distribute everything on the prepared salad. Serve immediately.

Nutritional information / 1 serving

- Calories   393 Kcal
- carbohydrates 13 g
- Fiber   3 g
- Proteins   54 g
- fat   15 g

RAW LIME AVOCADO CAKE

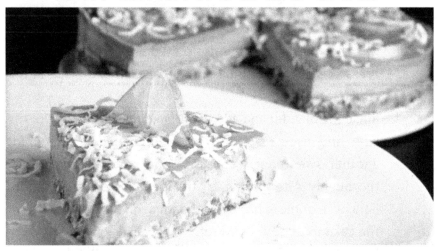

Ingredients for 8 servings

- 1/2 cup of dates
- 1 cup of almonds (I recommend this one)
- 1 cup of cashew nuts (I recommend this one)
- 1/2 cup desiccated coconut
- 3 avocados
- 2 bananas
- Juice and zest from 3 limes
- 4 tbsp honey

Preparation

Preparation 15 minutes

1. Mix the nuts, dates and desiccated coconut in a blender. Press the resulting dough into a cake tin and place in the refrigerator.
2. Rinse the blender and add the remaining ingredients for the lime and avocado foam: avocado, bananas, honey (or another sweetener), lime juice and zest. Mix everything thoroughly. After mixing, try the foam and either add more lime juice or more honey - depending on whether you want the cake to be sour or sweet.
3. Now apply the foam to the prepared dough. Put the cake in the refrigerator for the whole night or for at least 8 hours. Before serving, you can decorate the cake with lime or desiccated coconut.

Nutritional information / 1 slice

- Calories   375 Kcal
- carbohydrates 25 g
- Fiber   7 g
- Proteins   8 g
- fat   27 g

SWEET CHICKPEA DICE

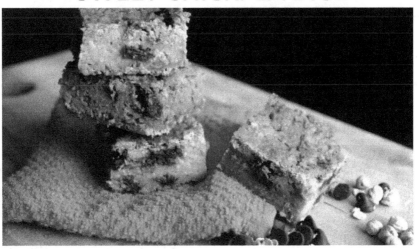

Ingredients for 16 servings

- 250 g of chickpeas (when dry) or 500 g of cooked chickpeas
- 1 cup of oatmeal (I recommend this one)
- 1/4 cup unsweetened applesauce
- 1 - 1.5 cups of honey
- 3 tbsp oil (coconut oil or other) (I recommend this one)
- Chocolate chips 70% or higher (to taste)
- Raisins / dried fruit / nuts (optional)
- 2 tsp vanilla extract
- 1/2 teaspoon of soda
- 2 teaspoons of baking soda
- 1/8 tsp sea salt

Preparation

Preparation 50 minutes

1. Grind the oat flakes or mix them finely. Mix all ingredients with the exception of the chocolate chips (or dried fruit and nuts) in a bowl. Divide the mixture into two (or more) parts and then mix them in the mixer. However, not in a large kitchen mixer, because the mass is too dry for that, but in a small chopper, which is available as an accessory for the hand blender. If you don't have it, try the hand blender.

2. When the whole mixture is completely mixed and smoothly mixed, add the chocolate chips (possibly also dried fruit and nuts).

3. Put the dough in a smaller baking pan / casserole dish / cake tin. The shape size is to be selected according to the desired thickness of the cake. However, I recommend that the cake is about 3 - 4 cm thick, it tastes better then.

4. Bake the cake for 35 - 40 minutes at 180 degrees (check again and again so that it does not burn).

5. Then let the cake cool down and put it in the fridge for one night, because the next day it tastes even better. Store in the refrigerator.

Nutritional information / 1 slice

- Calories   125 Kcal
- carbohydrates 23 g
- Fiber   2 g
- Proteins   2 g
- fat   3

Healthy piña colada

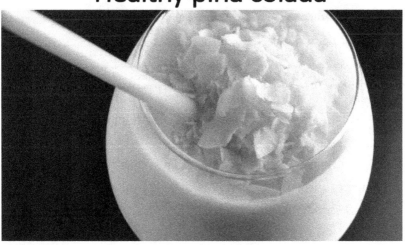

Ingredients for 4 servings

- 1 can of coconut milk (full fat content)
- 2 cans of pineapple in its own juice (or 500 g fresh pineapple)
- 1 cup of ice cubes
- Desiccated coconut for sprinkling

Preparation

Preparation 7 minutes

1. Mix all ingredients with the exception of the desiccated coconut in the mixer for approx. 30 seconds.
2. Serve the piña colada immediately after mixing.
3. Sprinkle with desiccated coconut or decorate with a piece of pineapple.
4. For the preparation of popsicle it is sufficient to distribute the prepared piña colada in popsicle molds and to put in the freezer for at least 2 hours.

Nutritional information / 1 serving

- Calories   245 Kcal
- carbohydrates 19 g
- Fiber   2 g
- Proteins   2 g
- fat   17 g

Sweet and sour lemon dessert without flour

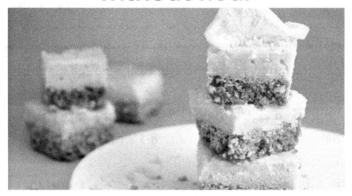

Ingredients for 10 servings

For the cake base:

- 1 cup of oatmeal (I recommend this one)
- 1/2 cup desiccated coconut
- 1 pinch of sea salt
- 1/2 teaspoon baking soda
- 1 egg
- 2 tbsp melted coconut oil (I recommend this one)
- 2 tbsp honey
- 3 tbsp applesauce

For the lemon filling:

- 3-4 tbsp honey
- 7 eggs
- Juice and zest of 4 lemons
- 2 tbsp corn starch

Preparation

Preparation 45 minutes

1. Grind the oatmeal and coconut to a fine flour.
2. Mix thoroughly with the rest of the dough ingredients in a bowl.
3. Pour the dough into a silicone mold or a cake pan lined with baking paper and bake for 8-10 minutes at 180 degrees Celsius until golden brown.
4. In a bowl, whisk the eggs with honey, cornstarch, lemon juice and lemon zest.
5. Pour the filling over the baked base and then bake again for 25 minutes at 150 degrees Celsius.
6. After baking, place the cake in the refrigerator for at least 4 hours so that the dessert can cool down properly.

Nutritional information / 1 slice

- Calories   183 Kcal
- carbohydrates 18 g
- Fiber   2 g
- Proteins   6 g
- fat   11 g

Healthy baked tuna balls

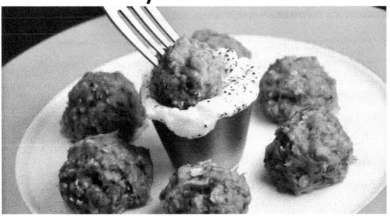

Ingredients for 1 serving

- 250 g tuna or salmon (canned or fresh)
- 20 g oatmeal (I recommend this one)
- 1 egg
- sea-salt
- ground pepper
- Garlic spice

Preparation

Preparation 25 minutes

1. Finely grind or chop the oatmeal.
2. Then knead in a bowl together with the tuna or salmon (juicing the canned fish), egg and spices to a mass according to taste.
3. Shape the dough into balls and spread them on the baking sheet lined with baking paper.
4. Bake the balls for 20 minutes at 180 degrees.
5. Serve the finished balls warm, preferably with yoghurt, dill or tomato sauce.

Nutritional information / 1 serving

- Calories 350 Kcal
- carbohydrates 12 g
- Fiber 2 g
- Proteins 57 g
- fat 7 g

Fitness Chicken Cake

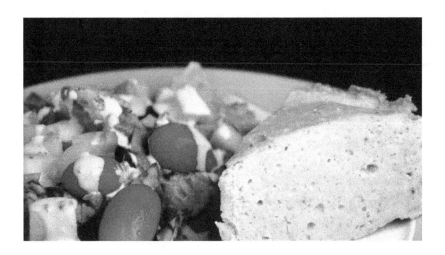

Ingredients for 4 servings

- 1 kg of chicken breast
- 100 g oatmeal (I recommend this one)
- 3 eggs
- 1 onion
- 1 teaspoon sea salt
- 1/2 teaspoon ground pepper
- 1/2 teaspoon garlic seasoning

Preparation

Preparation 50 minutes

1. Mix the oatmeal into flour in a mixer.
2. Add eggs, raw, diced chicken breast, sliced onion and spices and puree everything together thoroughly to form a smooth batter.
3. Pour the dough into a baking dish or a silicone bread box and bake for 40 - 45 minutes at 180 degrees until golden brown.

Nutritional information / 1 serving

- Calories   295 Kcal
- carbohydrates 6 g
- Fiber   1 g
- Proteins   51 g
- fat   5 g

Light grape salad with sour cream

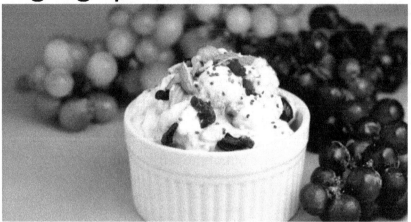

Ingredients for 4 servings

- 300 g of green and red grapes
- 100 g fresh blueberries
- 3 tbsp natural Greek yogurt
- 3 tbsp low-fat sour cream
- 30 g dried cranberries / raisins
- 40 g walnuts / pecans / almonds (I recommend these)
- 1 tbsp chia seeds (I recommend these)
- 1 vanilla pod (or 1/2 teaspoon vanilla extract)

Preparation

Preparation 15 minutes

1. Mix the yogurt with the sour cream in a bowl.
2. Stir in various seeds and kernels such as vanilla seeds, chia seeds, nuts, dried cranberries and others.
3. Finally add the washed grapes and blueberries.
4. The salad tastes good immediately after preparation or later when it comes out of the refrigerator.

Nutritional information / 1 serving

- Calories   157 Kcal
- carbohydrates 17 g
- Fiber   4 g
- Proteins   5 g
- fat   7 g

Sporty vegetable noodle salad with tuna

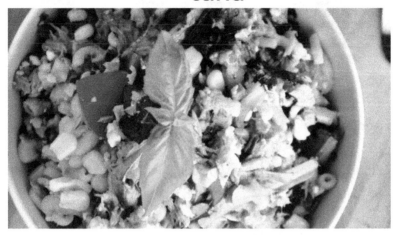

Ingredients for 2 servings

- 100 g whole wheat pasta (I recommend this one)
- 150 g tuna (in its own juice or olive oil)
- 2 handfuls of lettuce (garden, mixed salad, spring salad ...)
- 1 tomato
- 80 g corn
- 2 tbsp olive oil
- 4 tbsp cottage cheese (or more)
- Olives (optional)
- 1 pinch of sea salt
- Black pepper or other spices (to taste)

Preparation

Preparation 25 minutes

1. Cook the pasta in salted, boiling water according to the package instructions.
2. Rinse, finely chop the lettuce and tomato and place in a bowl.
3. Then mix in the corn, quark and olive oil.
4. Add the cooked pasta and drained tuna and stir the salad thoroughly.
5. Finally, season the vegetable salad with pepper and sea salt to taste.

Nutritional information / 1 serving

- Calories   449 Kcal
- carbohydrates 43 g
- Fiber   7 g
- Proteins   28 g
- fat   17 g

Healthy cocoa ice cream

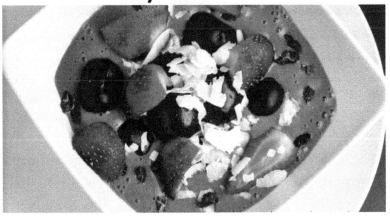

Ingredients for 2 servings

- 2 - 3 ripe bananas
- 4 tbsp cocoa (I recommend this one)
- 3 tbsp (Greek) yogurt

Preparation

Preparation 5 minutes

1. Freeze the cut bananas for a day or at least 4 hours. Take out of the freezer, put in the blender and add cocoa and (preferably Greek) yoghurt. Blend until you have a thick ice cream. Serve the ice cream right away. I recommend enriching it with fruit, cocoa beans or desiccated coconut.

2. The thicker the ice cream should be, the more frozen bananas should be added. If you want to sweeten it further, I recommend adding some dates. Put any leftover ice in the freezer and take it out a few minutes before you eat it again. Add other fruit and possibly peanut butter or quark and you can look forward to new taste experiences.

Nutritional information / 1 serving

- Calories   148 Kcal
- carbohydrates 27 g
- Fiber   7 g
- Proteins   6 g
- fat   3 g

Apple protein cheesecake bars

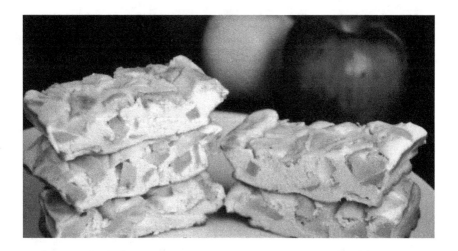

Ingredients for 5 servings

- 1 larger apple
- 2 eggs
- 170 g Greek yogurt
- 30 g protein powder (preferably vanilla protein powder, sweetened with stevia) (I recommend this one)
- some cinnamon

Preparation

Preparation 50 minutes

1. Cut the apples into small cubes and fry them dry in the pan with a pinch of cinnamon (approx. 3 minutes).
2. Mix yoghurt, eggs and protein powder together well in a bowl.
3. If you're not using sweetened protein powder, add a little stevia to the batter to taste.
4. Now stir in the fried apples and pour the dough into the bread box lined with baking paper (or another shape).
5. If you use a silicone mold, you don't need parchment paper.
6. Bake the dough for 40 minutes at 180 degrees. After baking, let the dough cool down, then take it out of the mold and cut it.

Nutritional information / 1 slice

- Calories   87 Kcal
- carbohydrates 6 g
- Fiber   1 g
- Proteins   10 g
- fat   3 g

Fitness salad with tuna, peas and cheese

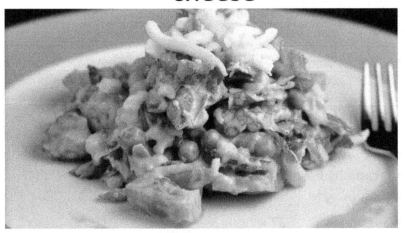

Ingredients for 2 servings

- 150 g tuna in olive oil
- 100 g Greek plain yogurt
- 100 g peas
- 50 g corn
- 40 g grated cheese (mozzarella)
- 2 handfuls of lettuce
- 5 pickles
- 1 tomato
- 1 tbsp mustard
- 1 tbsp ketchup (sugar-free)
- 1 clove of garlic

Preparation

Preparation 15 minutes

1. Wash the lettuce under running water and then finely chop it.
2. Mix thoroughly with the other ingredients in a bowl.
3. The salad tastes best immediately after preparation.

Nutritional information / 1 serving

- Calories   326 Kcal
- carbohydrates 19 g
- Fiber   5 g
- Proteins   37 g
- fat   10 g

Healthy tuna salad with beetroot and nuts

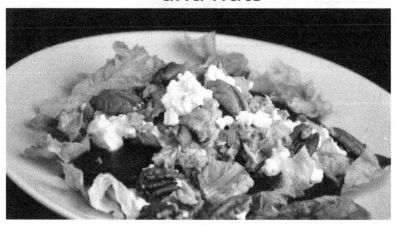

Ingredients for 2 servings

- 2 handfuls of lettuce or baby spinach
- 200 g cooked, sliced beetroot (or canned)
- 100 g of cottage cheese or goat cheese
- 150 g tuna in olive oil
- 2 tbsp lemon juice
- 40 g nuts (pecans, walnuts, etc.) (I recommend these)
- ground pepper

Preparation

Preparation 8 minutes

1. In a bowl, mix the tuna with oil, lemon juice, ground pepper and finely chopped lettuce / spinach.
2. Add beetroot, cottage cheese and nuts and serve.

Nutritional information / 1 serving

- Calories   390 Kcal
- carbohydrates 11 g
- Fiber   5 g
- Proteins   37 g
- fat   21 g

Light zucchini fruit salad with lime sauce

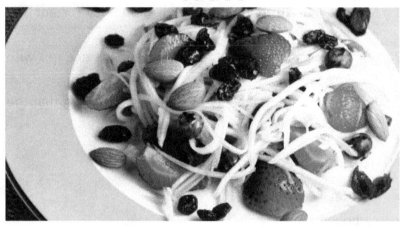

Ingredients for 2 servings

1. 1 large zucchini
2. 200 g strawberries
3. 100 g blueberries
4. 50 g dry cranberries / raisins
5. 40 g almonds (I recommend this one)
6. Juice from 1 lime
7. 1 tbsp honey

Preparation

Preparation 8 minutes

1. Mix the lime juice in a bowl with the honey (or another sweetener).
2. Cut the zucchini into pasta or another shape and mix with the lime sauce.
3. Add the other ingredients and mix well again so that the flavors combine.

Nutritional information / 1 serving

- Calories   202 Kcal
- carbohydrates 20 g
- Fiber   6 g
- Proteins   7 g
- fat   10 g

Quinoa in guacamole

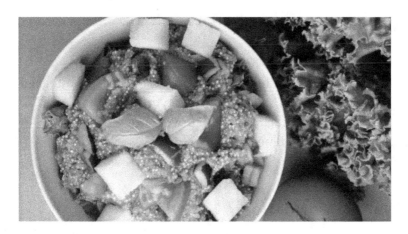

Ingredients for 2 servings

- 1 avocado
- 1 tomato (or 5 cherry tomatoes)
- Juice from 1 lime
- 1/2 cup quinoa (dry)
- 1 clove of garlic
- 150 g pineapple / mango
- salad
- some parsley
- 1/4 red onion
- 1 pinch of ground pepper
- 1 pinch of sea salt

Preparation

Preparation 15 minutes

1. Boil the quinoa with 1 cup of water.
2. Mash the avocado in a bowl and add lime juice, squeezed garlic, pepper and salt and mix everything well.
3. Now add the remaining finely chopped ingredients.
4. Serve the salad immediately or chilled.

Nutritional information / 1 serving

- Calories   341 Kcal
- carbohydrates 41 g
- Fiber   9 g
- Proteins   9 g
- fat   14 g

Healthy Tuna Sandwich

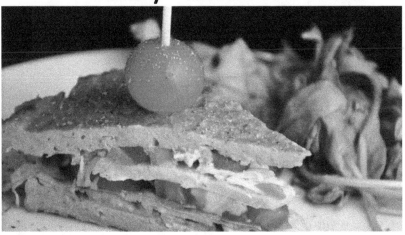

Ingredients for 2 servings

- 120 g of tuna in its own juice
- 1 egg
- 3 tbsp whole meal flour (or chickpea flour)
- Garlic spice
- ground pepper
- red pepper powder
- sea-salt

Preparation

Preparation 20 minutes

1. Juice the tuna and stir thoroughly with the egg and 3 spoons of flour.
2. Season to taste with spices and salt.
3. Pour the batter into a small baking pan or a baking dish lined with baking paper.
4. The dough is to be spread over the entire surface.
5. It becomes quite dense, so it is sufficient to distribute it in a square about 0.5 cm high.
6. Bake for 10-15 minutes at 180 degrees until golden brown.
7. Halve the finished sandwich dough, fill it as required and cut it diagonally.

Nutritional information / 1 serving

- Calories   135 Kcal
- carbohydrates 8 g
- Fiber   2 g
- Proteins   17 g
- fat   4 g

Almond coconut biscuits filled with banana ice cream

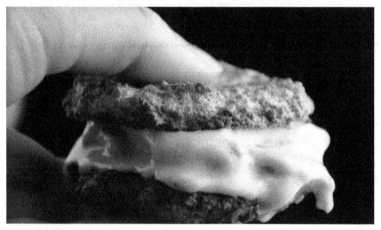

Ingredients for 4 servings

- 100 g almond flour
- 30 g desiccated coconut
- 3 egg whites
- 1 - 2 tbsp honey
- 3 bananas

Preparation

Preparation 30 minutes

1. Place the bananas cut in circles in the freezer for at least 8 hours.
2. Beat the egg whites in a bowl and then add the almond flour, desiccated coconut and honey (or another sweetener).
3. Gently stir the dough and place with a spoon on a baking sheet lined with baking paper.
4. The batter should make 10 cookies.
5. Bake the cookies brownish for about 20 minutes at 200 degrees.
6. Let the finished biscuits cool down and then fill them with banana ice cream.
7. Making the ice cream: Mix the frozen bananas in the food processor.

Nutritional information / 1 serving

- Calories   238 Kcal
- carbohydrates 20 g
- Fiber   5 g
- Proteins   8 g
- fat   14 g

Healthy broccoli salad with cottage cheese, tuna and corn

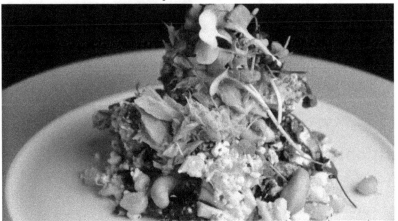

Ingredients for 2 servings

- 200 g raw broccoli
- 250 g of cottage cheese
- 80 g corn
- 1 handful of lettuce (garden, salad mix ...)
- 30 g cashew nuts (I recommend this one)
- 1-2 cloves of garlic
- fresh basil (to taste)
- 1 pinch of sea salt
- 1 pinch of black pepper (ground)
- 1 pinch of ginger powder
- 150 g tuna in its own juice

Preparation

Preparation 15 minutes

1. Cut the cleaned raw broccoli into fine pieces.
2. Mix the curd, spices, corn and chopped garlic in a bowl.
3. Add broccoli and salt to taste.
4. To increase the protein content, I recommend serving the salad together with tuna in its own juice.

Nutritional information / 1 serving

- Calories   360 Kcal
- carbohydrates 25 g
- Fiber   4 g
- Proteins   48 g
- fat   9 g

Beef rolls with prunes

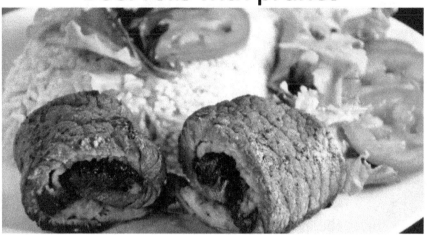

Ingredients for 2 servings

- 2 beef steaks
- 4 - 6 pieces of prunes
- 2 slices of bacon (or ham)
- 1 tbsp olive oil
- onion
- sea-salt
- pepper
- For the sauce:
- 1 tbsp chickpea flour
- 5 tbsp milk
- pepper

Preparation

Preparation 40 minutes

1. Knock the beef steaks. Then season with salt and pepper. Place bacon / ham and a few prunes on each steak and roll up. Fix each roll with a roulade needle.
2. Now lightly fry the onion with a little oil in a steam pot or a deep pan. Add the prepared rolls and pour water over them. Steam the rolls for about 30 minutes until tender. Check from time to time whether there is still enough water in the pot. Refill if necessary.
3. Get the finished rolls out of the pot. For the sauce, mix the milk, chickpea flour and pepper. Bring the sauce to the boil and pour it over the rolls. Serve with brown rice and vegetables.

Nutritional information / 1 serving

- Calories   315 Kcal
- carbohydrates 12 g
- Fiber   2 g
- Proteins   35 g
- fat   13 g

Marzipan fruit basket

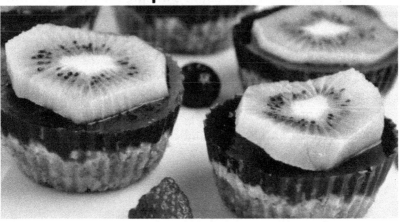

Ingredients for 6 servings

- 150 g almonds (preferably without the shell) (I recommend this)
- 2 tbsp honey
- 1 tbsp melted coconut oil (I recommend this one)
- 200 g fruit (strawberries, raspberries, blueberries etc.)
- 4 tbsp water
- 2 tbsp 100% gelatin powder
- 1 tbsp honey (optional)

Preparation

Preparation 15 minutes

1. Mix the almonds, melted coconut oil and honey (or any other liquid sweetener) together thoroughly in a blender. Press the resulting marzipan mixture onto the bottom of the silicone baskets or other silicone molds and place in the freezer.

2. Now prepare the fruit overflow: Boil the fruit with the water in a saucepan for about 3 minutes and then mix with a hand mixer or mash with a fork. Add the gelatin powder and possibly the sweetener to the fruit pulp and reheat everything. Remove from heat just before cooking.
3. Let the fruit mixture cool down briefly and then pour it onto the marzipan portion. Place the finished baskets in the refrigerator for at least 8 hours and decorate with fruit before consumption (optional).

Nutritional information / 1 serving

- Calories   186 kcal
- carbohydrates 9 g
- Fiber   4 g
- Proteins   6 g
- fat   14 g

Delicious zucchini casserole

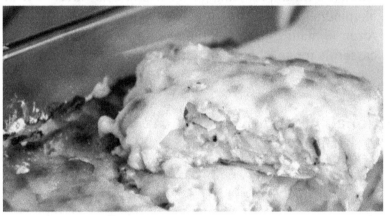

Ingredients for 4 servings

- 2 zucchinis (approx. 3.5 cups of grated zucchini)
- 2 eggs
- 1/2 teaspoon sea salt
- 1 teaspoon ground pepper
- 100 g grated cheese (mozzarella, parmesan, etc.)

Preparation

Preparation 50 minutes

1. Wash and grate the zucchini and then squeeze out the water by hand.
2. Mix the juiced zucchini in a bowl with eggs, salt, pepper and 2 spoons of cheese.
3. Put the resulting dough in a baking dish (e.g. 15 x 23 cm), sprinkle with the remaining cheese and bake covered with aluminum foil for 30 minutes at 190 degrees.
4. After 30 minutes, remove the aluminum foil and bake the casserole for another 15 minutes until golden brown.

Nutritional information / 1 slice

- Calories   110 kcal
- carbohydrates 3 g
- Fiber   1 g
- Proteins   10 g
- fat   7 g

Chinese style chicken breast

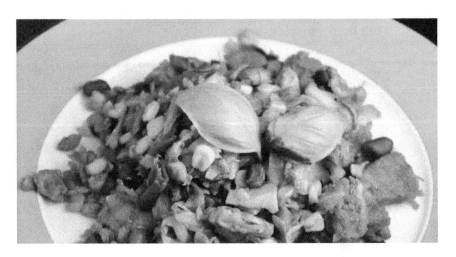

Ingredients for 4 servings

- 800 g of chicken
- 1 small cabbage
- 1 onion
- 250 g corn
- 200 g peas
- 250 g mushrooms
- 2 tbsp coconut oil (I recommend this one)
- 1 - 4 tbsp honey
- 5 tbsp soy sauce
- 1/2 teaspoon curry
- sea-salt
- Peanuts (optional)

Preparation

Preparation 40 minutes

1. Melt honey in a large saucepan over heated oil to a foam. If you like sweeter Chinese food, I recommend adding more than 1 spoonful of honey. When the honey starts to foam, add the chicken breast cut into noodles, stir occasionally and fry until pink for 10-20 minutes.
2. When the juice has completely evaporated, add the soy sauce and noodle cabbage to the meat and steam until the cabbage is cooked through. Then add the cut mushrooms, curry, peas and corn. Finally add the finely chopped onion, but do not fry anymore, just mix. Try and, if necessary, season with sea salt. Finally, you can add unroasted peanuts.

Serve the finished dish with rice or couscous, bulgur, quinoa or straight.

Nutritional information / 1 serving

- Calories   460 Kcal
- carbohydrates 28 g
- Fiber   9 g
- Proteins   56 g
- fat   10 g

Stuffed zucchini with tuna from the oven

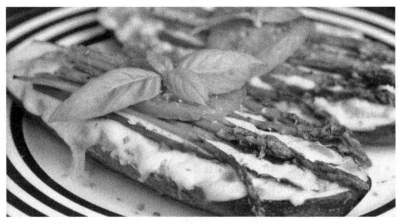

Ingredients for 1 serving

- 1 small zucchini
- 150 g tuna in its own juice
- 1/8 onion
- 1/2 teaspoon sweet paprika (ground)
- 1/4 tbsp salt
- oregano
- 1 clove of garlic
- 2 tsp mustard
- 3 tbsp Greek yogurt
- 50 g asparagus
- 30 g grated mozzarella
- 50 g smoked tofu (optional)

Preparation

Preparation 30 minutes

1. Wash the zucchini, cut off the stem and cut in half lengthways.
2. Scoop out the inside of the zucchini with a spoon. The pulp can be used for other recipes.
3. Place the zucchini boats in a baking dish or on a baking sheet.
4. In a bowl, mix the drained tuna with pepper, salt, yogurt, mustard, finely chopped onions and the crushed clove of garlic. Add the smoked tofu if you like.
5. Mix the ingredients thoroughly and distribute them on the prepared zucchini boats.
6. Place the cleaned asparagus on top and sprinkle with cheese.
7. Bake at 205 degrees Celsius for about 20 minutes.
8. The finished zucchini should be nice and soft, but not fall apart.

Nutritional information / 1 serving

- Calories   220 kcal
- carbohydrates 7 g
- Fiber   2 g
- Proteins   43 g
- fat   2 g

Healthy zucchini pizza dough

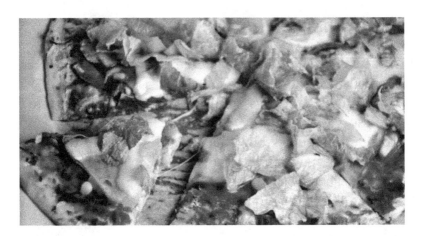

Ingredients for 2 servings

- 1 zucchini
- 2 eggs
- 50-100 g grated cheese
- sea-salt
- ground pepper
- Garlic spice

Preparation

Preparation 30 minutes

1. Grate the zucchini and squeeze out as much juice as possible by hand or with a towel.
2. Then mix with the eggs, spices, salt (to taste) and the grated cheese.
3. Decide for yourself how much cheese you like - the pizza tastes great even with 50 g cheese, but it becomes even more delicious and firm with 100 g cheese.
4. Spread the finished dough on the baking sheet lined with baking paper and bake for 15 minutes at 190 degrees.
5. Then cover with ingredients of your choice and bake for another 10 minutes.

Nutritional information / 1 serving

- Calories   142 Kcal
- carbohydrates 3 g
- Fiber   1 g
- Proteins   13 g
- fat   9 g

The best healthy avocado egg salad

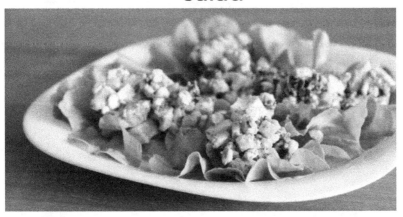

Ingredients for 2 servings

- 4 eggs
- 1 ripe avocado
- 200 g of cottage cheese
- 40 g corn
- 30 g dried tomatoes
- 1 pinch of salt
- 1 pinch of garlic powder
- 1 pinch of black pepper (ground)
- Spring onion
- Lettuce leaves

Preparation

Preparation 25 minutes

1. First prepare the hard-boiled eggs (put them in boiling water for about 8 minutes).
2. Let cool, peel, cut into small pieces and place in a bowl.
3. Then mix the cleaned and finely chopped avocado, spring onions, cottage cheese, sundried tomatoes, corn, salt and pepper with the eggs.
4. Stir the salad well and season to taste if necessary.
5. Fill onto a large leaf of lettuce to serve.

Nutritional information / 1 serving

- Calories   400 kcal
- carbohydrates 16 g
- Fiber   8 g
- Proteins   28 g
- fat   24 g

Zucchini spagetti with tuna sauce

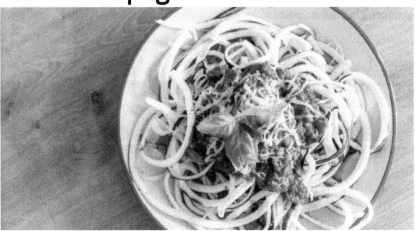

Ingredients for 2 servings

- 2 small zucchinis
- 150-200 g of tuna in its own juice
- 4 - 5 tbsp tomato paste
- 4 tbsp water
- 40 g of grated cheese
- pepper
- basil
- sea-salt

Preparation

Preparation 15 minutes

1. Wash the zucchini and peel the spaghetti with a peeler. If you don't have a peeler, you can just rub it on the rasp.
2. Mix the tomato paste in a saucepan with a few spoons of water (the amount of water determines how thick the sauce will be).
3. When the consistency of the sauce is desired, add the tuna, season with pepper and cook the sauce.
4. Bring to the boil and then pour over the zucchini spagetti.
5. I recommend topping the dish with cheese and fresh basil at the end.

Nutritional information / 1 serving

- Calories   161 Kcal
- carbohydrates 8 g
- Fiber   3 g
- Proteins   23 g
- fat   5 g

Healthy, sweet chickpea pulp

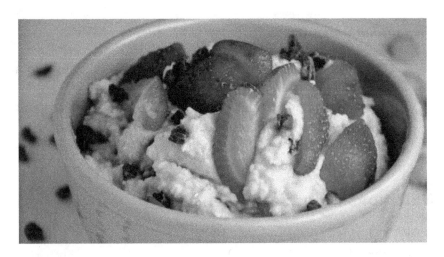

Ingredients for 2 servings

- 1/4 cup applesauce (or peanut / almond butter) (I recommend this)
- 1/4 cup milk (of your choice)
- 3 tbsp oatmeal (I recommend this one)
- 2 tbsp honey
- 1 pinch of salt
- 1 scoop of protein powder (optional) (I recommend this one)
- Fruit, dark chocolate (70% or higher), cocoa beans, raisins, nuts, desiccated coconut (optional)
- 1.5 cups (250 g) cooked chickpeas

Preparation

Preparation 5 minutes

1. Put the chickpeas, applesauce, milk, oatmeal, honey and a pinch of salt in the blender and puree until smooth.
2. Tip: add protein powder - if it is flavored, adjust the amount of honey (or the sweetener used instead) to suit your taste.
3. Stir fruit, dark chocolate, cocoa beans or raisins into the smooth pulp and serve.

Nutritional information / 1 serving

- Calories   176 Kcal
- carbohydrates 35 g
- Fiber   4 g
- Proteins   5 g
- fat   1 g

CONCLUSIONS

Dairy-free diet is justified in people with intolerances, avoiding dairy products and buying Dairy-free foods often sounds like a healthy lifestyle - but is not necessary for many people. Only between 25 and 40% of people suffer from lactose intolerance and should therefore avoid certain foods in order not to be constantly plagued by stomach problems. But doing without lactose does not only mean avoiding dairy products, because milk sugar is also hidden in completely different foods.

There are no adverse effects from stopping Dairy as long as the nutrients they provide are replaced. Dairy is a sugar (disaccharide) that can cause intolerances. Dairy and wheat are restricted in low-FODMAP diets. Now it is worth clarifying that these diets are not to be consumed for a long time. When Dairy is eliminated from the diet for a long time, it is digested less and less. The body stops "making" lactase and intolerance appears. In these cases, free milks indicated Dairy or milk "predigested" as yogurt. Yogurt contains 30% less Dairy than milk. The Dairy in yogurt has been fermented by lactic bacteria that convert it into lactic acid.